Introduction to the Masticatory System and Dental Occlusion

Dinesh Rokaya

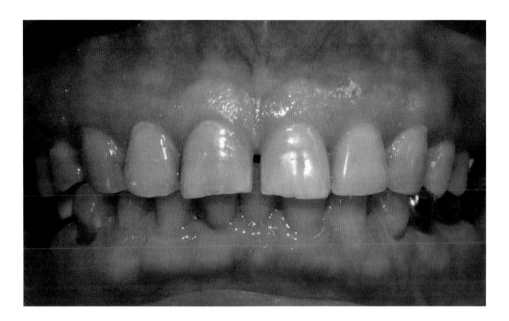

Introduction to the Masticatory System and Dental Occlusion

Dinesh Rokaya, PhD
Clinical Sciences Department
College of Dentistry
Ajman University
Ajman, United Arab Emirates

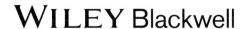

Registered Offices
John Wiley & Sons, Inc., 111 River Street, Hoboken, NJ 07030, USA
John Wiley & Sons Ltd, The Atrium, Southern Gate, Chichester, West Sussex, PO19 8SQ, UK

For details of our global editorial offices, customer services, and more information about Wiley products visit us at www.wiley.com.

Wiley also publishes its books in a variety of electronic formats and by print-on-demand. Some content that appears in standard print versions of this book may not be available in other formats.

Library of Congress Cataloging-in-Publication Data
Names: Rokaya, Dinesh, author.
Title: Introduction to the masticatory system and dental occlusion / Dinesh Rokaya.
Description: Hoboken, NJ : Wiley Blackwell, 2025. | Includes bibliographical references and index.
Identifiers: LCCN 2023043797 (print) | LCCN 2023043798 (ebook) | ISBN 9781119884187 (paperback) | ISBN 9781119884194 (adobe pdf) | ISBN 9781119884200 (epub)
Subjects: MESH: Stomatognathic System–anatomy & histology | Dental Occlusion | Stomatognathic Diseases
Classification: LCC RK523 (print) | LCC RK523 (ebook) | NLM WU 101 | DDC 617.6/43–dc23/eng/20231106
LC record available at https://lccn.loc.gov/2023043797
LC ebook record available at https://lccn.loc.gov/2023043798

Cover Design: Wiley
Cover Images: © Dinesh Rokaya

Set in 9.5/12.5pt STIXTwoText by Straive, Pondicherry, India
Printed in Singapore
M121188_181024

Dedication

This text is personally dedicated to the memory of my grandfather Mr. Singh Bir Rokaya, my father Mr. Jaya Bahadur Rokaya, my aunt Mrs. Laxmi Sharma and my brother-in-law Mr. Aadhi Kathayat and dedicated to all my family members, advisors, and friends for their help, support, and encouragement.

Contents

About the Author

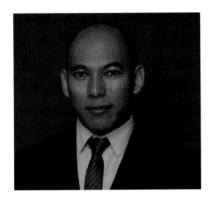

Dinesh Rokaya received a Bachelor of Dental Surgery from People's Dental College and Hospital affiliated with Tribhuvan University, Nepal in 2009 and Master of Science in Dentistry in Maxillofacial Prosthetics from the Faculty of Dentistry, Mahidol University, Thailand in 2015, and Doctor of Philosophy in Dental Biomaterials Science from Faculty of Dentistry, Chulalongkorn University, Thailand in 2019. He then did a one-year Postdoctoral Fellowship in Dental Biomaterials from the Faculty of Dentistry, Chulalongkorn University, Thailand (2019–2020). He is a registered prosthodontist and dental biomaterials specialist in Nepal Medical Council. He has also received a Diploma of Membership of the Faculty of Dental Surgery (MFDS) from the Royal College of Surgeons of England and the Royal College of Physicians and Surgeons of Glasgow. He is also a Fellow of the Higher Education Academy (FHEA), UK and an Affiliate Fellow of the American Academy of Maxillofacial Prosthetics (AAMP), USA. He has co-authored over 115 articles in international peer-reviewed journals and 15 book chapters (H-index 28). He is an Assistant Professor at the Clinical Sciences Department, College of Dentistry, Ajman University, Ajman, United Arab Emirates. He is also a Visiting Professor at the Department of Prosthodontics, Faculty of Dentistry, Chulalongkorn University, Bangkok, Thailand. His research areas include prosthetic dentistry, digital dentistry, esthetic dentistry, and dental biomaterials. He is a member of the American Dental Association, British Society of Prosthodontics, International College of Prosthodontics, International Association of Dental Research, International Society of Maxillofacial Rehabilitation, and International Association of Dental Research. He is a life member of the Nepal Dental Association and Nepal Medical Association.

Foreword

As a prosthodontist at Chulalongkorn University, Thailand, I am delighted to see the book "Masticatory System and Dental Occlusion" written by Dr. Dinesh Rokaya which is published by Wiley Publications. The masticatory system and occlusion in dentistry are important subjects for both undergraduate and postgraduate dental students. Although masticatory system and occlusion can sometimes seem to be difficult to understand, the contents in this book clarify them and make them easier to understand. This book describes the anatomic features that are fundamental to comprehending the dental anatomy, masticatory system, temporomandibular joint, muscles of mastication, and dental occlusion. This also covers the problems in occlusion and treatment options. Lastly, I would like to congratulate Dr. Dinesh Rokaya for his hard work in contributing such a valuable book. This book will not only be a benefit to dental students but also to anyone who wants to learn masticatory system and occlusion.

Associate Prof. Viritpon Srimaneepong
Department of Prosthodontics
Faculty of Dentistry, Chulalongkorn University
Bangkok 10400, Thailand

Foreword 2

Masticatory science and dental occlusion are important topics in dentistry. Understanding the functional anatomy in dentistry is essential to the study of dental occlusion. The knowledge of the masticatory system and dental occlusion is used in various aspects of clinical dentistry such as restorative dentistry, prosthodontics, orthodontics, oral and maxillofacial surgery. I believe that the book "Masticatory System and Dental Occlusion" written by Dr. Dinesh Rokaya is useful for undergraduate dental students.

Finally, I would like to congratulate Dr. Dinesh Rokaya for his contribution and hard work in making this book successful.

Associate Prof. Ahmad Al Jaghsi
Clinical Sciences Department, College of Dentistry
Center of Medical and Bio-Allied Health Sciences Research
Head, Continuing Education Office and Staff Development
Head of Cellular and Material Sciences Research Group
Ajman University, Ajman, United Arab Emirates

Visiting Associate Professor
Department of Prosthodontics, Gerodontology, and Dental Materials
Greifswald University Medicine, 17489 Greifswald, Germany

Foreword 3

The topic of masticatory science and dental occlusion is always confusing to dental students. Understanding the functional anatomy and biomechanics in dentistry is essential to the study of dental occlusion. The knowledge of the masticatory system and dental occlusion can be applied in restorative dentistry, prosthodontics, periodontics, and oral and maxillofacial surgery. I believe that this book is very useful for undergraduates in dentistry. This book describes the anatomic features that are basic to an understanding of the masticatory system and dental occlusion. The contents of this book include basic dental anatomy, temporomandibular joints, muscles of mastication, and dental occlusion.

Finally, I would like to congratulate Dr. Dinesh Rokaya for his continuous effort in making this book project successful.

Prof. Sittichai Koontonkaew
Dean, Walailak University International College of Dentistry
Walailak University
Bangkok 10400, Thailand

Preface

Although the dentistry field is advancing and progressing, a sound understanding of functional dental anatomy and biomechanics is essential in every aspect of dentistry. This book describes the anatomic features that are basic to an understanding of the masticatory system and dental occlusion.

This book gathers and provides an introductory guide to the masticatory system and dental occlusion. This book has 11 chapters ranging from the anatomy of the masticatory system, tooth alignments, functions of the masticatory system, bruxism and clenching, nervous system regulating masticatory system, age changes of the masticatory system, occlusal concept and its application in various aspects of dentistry, and problems in dental occlusion and their treatments.

Although this book is useful for undergraduates in dentistry, such as BDS, DDS, DMD, DDent, BDent, BDSc, or BScD. Similarly, this book is also useful for students in dental hygiene, dental technology, and dental assistants. In addition, this book will be useful for recent graduates who want to keep updated in the field of dental occlusion and masticatory system. This book can be useful for graduates who are appearing in competitive dental exams for further dental education or dental license.

Dinesh Rokaya

Acknowledgments

I would never accomplish it on my own but rather represent the accumulation of many people. A lot of people have supported me for this book. First and foremost are Prof. Sittichai Koontonkaew and Prof. Natthamet Wongsirichat for their support and inspiration in writing this book. I would like to thank Dr. Dipendra K.C. for his encouragement for this book. I am grateful to Assoc. Prof. Dr. Viritpon Srimaneepong for his continued support and encouragement for this book. I would like to thank my uncle Mr. Anga Lal Rokaya for his encouragement. Finally, I am highly grateful to my brother Dr. Nabin Rokaya, and my wife Dr. Goma Kathayat, who helped me a lot in the editing of the chapters. I would also like to thank Dr. Sonica Khanal for the drawings and editing. I also thank Dr. Bishwa Prakash Bhattarai for his suggestions.

I am deeply grateful to the WILEY publication for accepting my proposal and publishing this book. I am deeply grateful to Mr. Selvakumar Gunakundru and Mr. Raj Oliver at Wiley for their guidance, coordination, and production of this book. I also want to express my appreciation to Mr. Atul Ignatius David and Ms. Susan Engelken and Mrs. Loan Nguyen for their support, guidance, and coordination of this book. I will also like to thank to many others at Wiley for their behind-the-scene works and contributions to this book.

Lastly, I am grateful to my family, advisors, colleagues, and friends who supported me. It does take a community for the completion of this textbook and I thank you all.

Dinesh Rokaya

1

Structures and Functions of Masticatory System

1.1 Introduction

The masticatory system consists of teeth, muscles, ligaments, bones, and joints, which are responsible for functions of the masticatory system, i.e. mastication, speech, swallowing, and speaking. The system also assists in breathing. It is regulated and coordinated by the neurologic controlling system. The musculature aids in specific motion of the mandible and effective teeth movement during function. To study occlusion, explicit knowledge of biomechanics and functional anatomy of mastication is crucial.

1.2 Structures and Functions of Temporomandibular Joint

The temporomandibular joints (TMJs) are synovial joints and movable articulations in the skull [1, 2]. The muscles of mastication along with the suprahyoid and infrahyoid move the TMJ and play a crucial part in jaw movements. The basic components of the TMJ include (Figures 1.1 and 1.2) the mandible (head of the condyle), disc, temporal bone (glenoid fossa and articular eminence), and the capsule surrounding the TMJs.

1.2.1 Articular Surfaces

Each TMJ is formed by the mandible's condylar head and squamous temporal bone's articular surfaces. Mostly, the synovial joints are shielded by the hyaline cartilage; however, the articular surfaces of TMJs are shielded by fibrocartilage (predominantly collagen accompanied by few chondrocytes), which makes them atypical [3, 4]. During jaw movements, the condyles translate forward onto the convex articular eminence.

1.2.2 Ligaments

The ligaments are mainly built from collagenous connective tissue fibers of distinct lengths. Normally, they are nonstretchable, but they can be elongated if extensive forces are applied. Ligaments control the movements of the border. The three major functional ligaments of

Introduction to the Masticatory System and Dental Occlusion, First Edition. Dinesh Rokaya.
© 2025 John Wiley & Sons Ltd. Published 2025 by John Wiley & Sons Ltd.

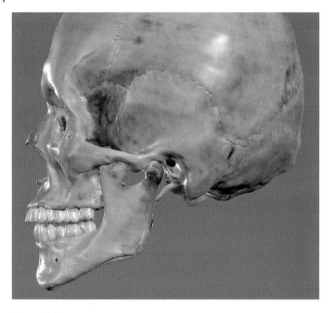

Figure 1.1 Left temporomandibular joint (TMJ) showing the condyle, disc, glenoid fossa, and articular eminence of the temporal bone. Image taken from the Anatomage Table (Anatomage Inc., California, USA).

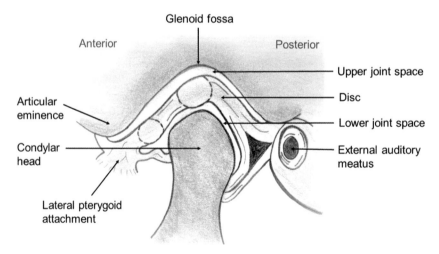

Figure 1.2 Diagram of the right temporomandibular joint (TMJ) sagittal section showing the various components.

the TMJ are the collateral, capsular, and temporomandibular ligaments (TMLs) [1, 5]. The accessory ligaments are two in number: sphenomandibular and stylomandibular.

1.2.2.1 Collateral (Discal) Ligaments
The other name for collateral ligaments is discal ligaments. These are the true ligaments that comprise fibers of collagenous connective tissue and are nonelastic. These ligaments divide

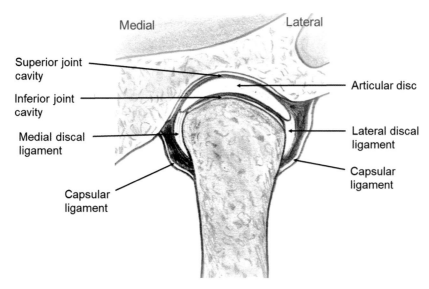

Figure 1.3 Anterior view of the temporomandibular joint (TMJ). Adapted from Reference [1]; chapter published in Management of Temporomandibular Disorders and Occlusion, 7th edition, Okeson J.P., Functional Anatomy and Biomechanics of the Masticatory System, page 10, Copyright Elsevier (2013).

the joint mediolaterally into the inferior and superior joint cavities. The articular disc (lateral and medial borders) is linked to the condyle by the collateral ligaments. The medial discal ligament connects the medial pole of the condyle from the medial edge of the disc, and the lateral discal ligament connects the lateral pole of the condyle from the lateral edge of the disc (Figure 1.3) [1]. During glides of the condyle anteriorly and posteriorly, passive movement with the condyle is permitted by them. Moreover, the anterior and posterior disc rotation on the condyle's articular surface is allowed by them. Hence, they are beneficial for the hinge motion of the TMJ that happens between the articular disc and the condyle.

1.2.2.2 Capsular Ligament
The capsular ligament incorporates the entire TMJ (Figure 1.4) [1]. Superiorly, the capsular ligament's fibers are connected to the temporal bone through the mandibular fossa's articular surfaces and the articular eminence. Inferiorly, the capsular ligament's fibers are connected to the condylar neck. The function of this ligament is to withstand all the forces arising medially, laterally, or inferiorly, which might result in the separation or dislocation of the articular surfaces. This ligament also helps retain the synovial fluid.

1.2.2.3 Temporomandibular Ligament
The strengthened capsular ligament builds the temporomandibular (TM) or the lateral ligament with the help of strong tight fibers. The TML consists of an inner horizontal portion and an outer oblique portion (Figure 1.4A) [1]. The inner horizontal portion stretches from the zygomatic process and articular tubercle horizontally to the condyle's lateral pole and the articular disc's posterior part. The outer oblique portion stretches from the articular tubercle and zygomatic process to the neck of the condyle.

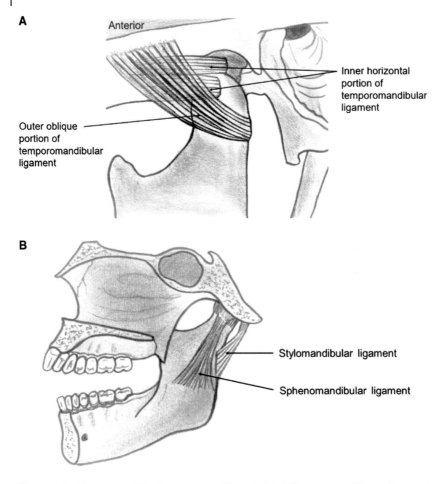

Figure 1.4 Ligaments of the temporomandibular joint. A, Temporomandibular ligament showing the outer oblique portion and the inner horizontal portion. B, Stylomandibular ligament and sphenomandibular ligament. Adapted from Reference [1]; chapter published in Management of Temporomandibular Disorders and Occlusion, 7th edition, Okeson J.P., Functional Anatomy and Biomechanics of the Masticatory System, page 10–11, Copyright Elsevier (2013).

1.2.2.4 Sphenomandibular Ligament

The sphenomandibular ligament is one of the accessory ligaments of the TMJ (Figure 1.4B) [1], which emerges from the sphenoid bone's spine and descends to the mandibular ramus' lingula [6]. This ligament has no crucial function in mandibular movement limitation.

1.2.2.5 Stylomandibular Ligament

The stylomandibular ligament is another accessory ligament of the TMJ (Figure 1.4B) [1], which emerges from the styloid process and descends downward and forward to the mandibular angle and posterior border of the ramus. The uncontrolled protrusive mandibular motions are limited by the stylomandibular ligament. This ligament becomes tense while protruding the mandible and relaxes while opening the mandible.

1.2.3 Nerve Innervation of the Temporomandibular Joint

The trigeminal nerve innervates the TMJ and supplies sensory and motor innervation to the muscles that regulate it. The afferent innervation is supplied by the mandibular nerve branches. Most of the innervation is supplied through the auriculotemporal nerve while it branches off the mandibular nerve. Masseteric and deep temporal nerves provide supplemental innervation [7].

1.2.4 Blood Supply of the Temporomandibular Joint

The principal arteries of the TMJs are composed of the middle meningeal artery anteriorly, the superficial temporal artery posteriorly, and the internal maxillary artery inferiorly. The deep auricular, ascending pharyngeal, and anterior tympanic arteries are the additional crucial vessels. The "feeder vessels" that by a direct route get into the head of the condyle both anteriorly and posteriorly and the inferior alveolar artery through marrow spaces are the routes through which the condyle acquires its vascular supply [8].

1.2.5 Functions of the Temporomandibular Joint

The function of the TMJ is based on the articular design, neuromuscular control, and integrity of soft tissue elements that comprise the anatomy [9]. The prime function of the TMJ is to facilitate movements of the lower jaw. This joint allows a range of movements of the lower jaw, i.e. translational movements (protrusion, retraction, and lateral deviation) and rotational movements (elevation and depression) [2, 9].

1.2.6 Clinical Evaluation of the Temporomandibular Joint

The clinical evaluation of the TMJ includes the observation of the symmetry of the face and the various movements of TMJ. In patients with TMJ dysfunction, it will result in an asymmetry of the mandibular branch.

Pain and clicking are recorded at specific degrees of articular opening or closing, along with accessory movements. The muscles are palpated (externally and internally) and the presence of enlarged submandibular lymph nodes is also checked by palpation. The jaw is slowly moved to evaluate the TMJ ligament apparatus. The fingers are placed on the joint while the patient opens his mouth to evaluate the TMJ. The maximum opening of the mouth should also be evaluated [10].

1.2.7 Radiographic Examination of the Temporomandibular Joint

Various instruments are used in the assessments of the TMJs, and they play a vital role in the diagnosis. Hence, it is necessary to do a proper assessment using instruments before taking a therapeutic approach to a TMJ in the dysfunction [11]. Various imaging techniques for the TMJ include panoramic radiography, plain radiography (transcranial projection), computed tomography or cone-beam computed tomography, and magnetic resonance imaging (Figure 1.5) [12–14]. Panoramic radiography (Figure 1.5A) is important in the

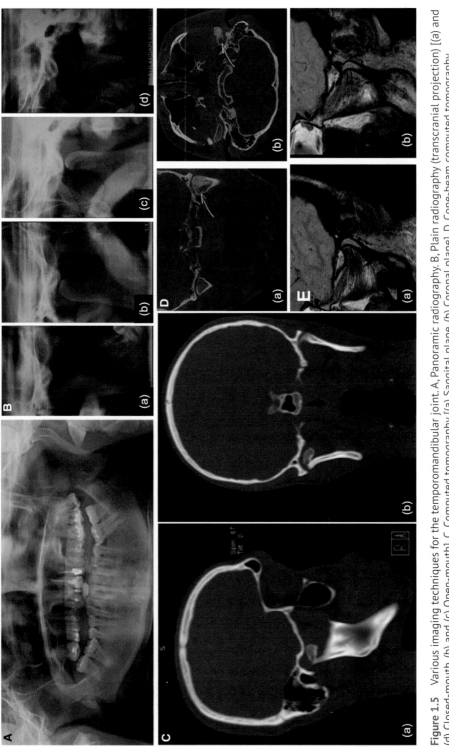

Figure 1.5 Various imaging techniques for the temporomandibular joint. A, Panoramic radiography. B, Plain radiography (transcranial projection) [(a) and (d) Closed-mouth, (b) and (c) Open-mouth]. C, Computed tomography [(a) Saggital plane, (b) Coronal plane]. D, Cone-beam computed tomography [(a) Coronal plane, (b) Axial plane]. E, Magnetic resonance imaging [(a) Closed-mouth, (b) Open-mouth]. Reproduced from [12] / with permission of Kathmandu University Medical Journal (KUMJ) Kathmandu University.

evaluation of the mandibular condyles to the glenoid fossa relationship. Plain radiography of the TMJs (Figure 1.5B) using transcranial projections is useful in the evaluation of the TMJ. The images can be taken at various angulations (lateral oblique transcranial projections, anterior–posterior projections, submental-vertex projection, transpharyngeal view) to avoid the superposition of the temporal bone and the opposite TMJ [13]. Computed tomography or cone-beam computed tomography (Figure 1.5C,D) is done to evaluate the morphology of the components that make up TMJ as well as bone position and pathologies [14]. Magnetic resonance imaging of TMJ (Figure 1.5E) helps observe the condition of the articular disk, anatomy, function, and form.

1.2.8 Clinical Considerations of the Temporomandibular Joint

Loss of teeth results in the subsequent loading of the TMJ, and it can lead to histomorphological and pathophysiological changes in the TMJ joint (the articular disc, articular cartilages, the synovium, and the articular bony components) [15]. The severity of the changes increases with increasing age and is aggravated by impaired occlusal stabilization and existing arthritis of the joint.

Various pathologies can affect the TMJ and potentially cause varying degrees of dysfunction [16]. Damage or disease in the joint area adversely affects masticatory function and speaking, affecting the quality of the life of the patient. Common conditions and diseases of the TMJ include joint pain, muscular pain, rheumatoid arthritis, ankylosing spondylitis, psoriatic arthropathy, fibromyalgia syndrome – myalgia, and multiple sclerosis.

Effective treatment options for patients suffering from severe TMJ disorders are in high demand because surgical options are restricted to the removal of damaged tissue or complete replacement of the joint with prosthetics. Surgical procedures for TMJ are performed for various medical reasons: local and/or systemic disease, trauma, alteration of joint morphology, and loss of function. The long-term outcome of TMJ arthroscopic surgery is acceptable and stable compared with other surgical procedures [17]. Total joint reconstruction using alloplastic joint replacement is done to treat the end-stage disease and has good post-surgical results in the presence of idiopathic condylar resorption [18].

1.3 Structures and Functions of Masticatory Muscles

Muscles are composed of several muscle fibers varying between 10 and 80 μm in diameter [1]. A single nerve ending innervates each fiber, which is situated close to the center of the fiber. The end part of the muscle fiber gathers into bundles forming the muscle tendon which inserts into the bone. Actin and myosin present in muscle fiber are polymerized proteins that have an important function in muscle contraction. Each one of the muscle fibers consists of several myofibrils. These myofibrils comprise approximately 3000 actin filaments and 1500 myosin filaments, situated side by side.

Based on the quantity of myoglobin pigment present in muscle fibers, they can be distinguished into two forms: Type I (slow) and Type II (fast) [19]. Type I fibers consist of a greater quantity of myoglobin and have a deep red color. They can maintain slow yet sustained contraction, are resistant to fatigue, and undergo aerobic metabolism. Type II fibers consist of less quantity of myoglobin and have a whiter color. They have a small number of mitochondria and depend more on anaerobic metabolism for activity. These fibers undergo rapid contraction; however, they fatigue quickly compared to slow fibers. A combination of slow and fast fibers is present in all the skeletal muscles in a diverse quantity that reflects the function of the muscle. Those muscles that must react promptly are mainly composed of white fibers. Slow fibers are present in those muscles that are chiefly utilized for continuous and slow activities. The primary muscles of mastication consist of four muscle pairs: temporalis, masseter, and medial and lateral pterygoids.

The features of masticatory muscles are that [20] (i) they develop from the mesoderm of the first pharyngeal arch, whereas the trunk and limb muscles develop from the somites; (ii) they have a wider range of myosin-heavy chains in adulthood, such as neonatal and cardiac isoforms; (iii) they have a greater number of hybrid fibers by which they have high force in a fatigue-resistant mode; (iv) their morphology of the fibers is unusual, with type II fibers smaller in diameter compared to type I; and (v) the velocity of shortening of their type I and type II fibers (slower and faster) as explained earlier [19, 21] and shown in Figure 1.6 [20]. In addition, the masticatory muscles are moldable based on environmental and genetic factors [21].

Besides, the jaws that are involved in mastication present some unique developmental and morphological features compared to the postcranial skeleton (the trunk and limbs) as shown in Figure 1.7) [20]. The features of the mandibular bone are that (i) they are developed from the embryonic neural crest cells instead of the embryonic mesoderm, (ii) they support teeth, (iii) they have some pathologies that are not present in other bones (some are related to the teeth), (iv) they contain more red bone marrow than yellow bone marrow, (v) their regeneration capacity is greater than that of the other bones, and (vi) they are under constant movement and mechanical loading from chewing, swallowing, and speech [22–25]. In addition, the muscle–bone functional relationship is involved in bone biomechanics, i.e. loading and movement affect its shape through the remodeling process [20].

The origin and insertion of various primary muscles of mastication (temporalis, masseter, and medial and lateral pterygoids) with their functions are shown in Table 1.1. Each of the muscles is discussed in detail, focusing on the direction, attachment, and function of the muscle fiber.

1.3.1 Temporalis

The temporalis is a broad fan-shaped muscle that emerges from the temporal fossa and the lateral surface of the skull. The temporalis fibers combine as they merge down between the zygomatic arch and the skull's lateral surface, making a tendon that inserts into the coronoid process and anterior border of the ramus of the mandible. The temporalis can be divided into three distinct areas (Figure 1.8A) [1]: the anterior portion (vertically directed fibers), the middle portion (obliquely directed fibers across the lateral surface of the skull), and the posterior portion (horizontally directed fibers running over the ear forward to merge with the other fibers of temporalis while they course below the zygomatic arch). The mandible is elevated as there is a contraction of the temporal muscle. Contraction of the anterior portion results in vertical elevation of the mandible, the middle portion results in

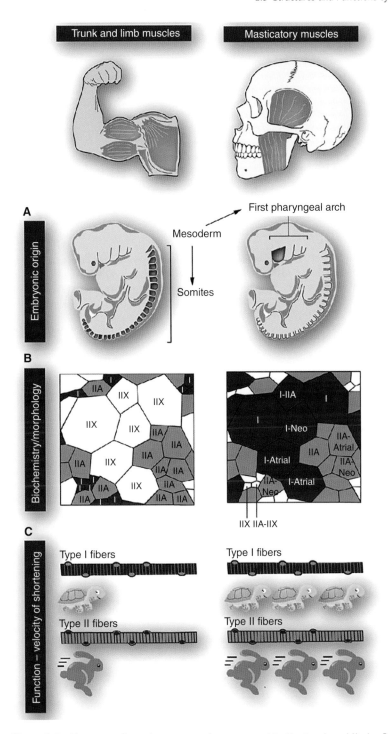

Figure 1.6 Features of masticatory muscles compared to the trunk and limbs. Reference [20] / Frontiers Media S.A. / CC BY 4.0.

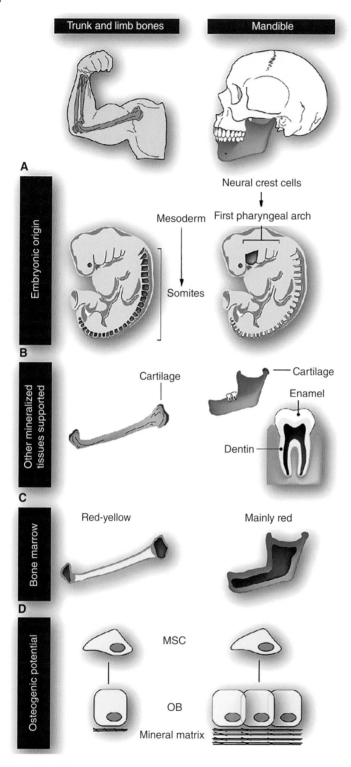

Figure 1.7 Features of mandibular bone compared to the trunk and limbs. Reference [20] / Frontiers Media S.A. / CC BY 4.0.

Table 1.1 Origin and insertion of various muscles of mastication.

Muscles	Origin	Insertion	Functions
Masseter	Zygomatic arch	Angle of the mandible Ramus of mandible	Closing the mouth Protrusion (superficial head) Retrusion (deep head) Ipsilateral excursion
Temporalis	Temporal fossa	Coronoid process Ramus of the mandible	Closing the mouth Retrusion (posterior fibers) Ipsilateral excursion
Medial pterygoid	Superficial head: maxillary tuberosity Deep head: Medial surface of the lateral pterygoid plate	Angle of the mandible Ramus of mandible	Closing the mouth Protrusion Contralateral excursion
Lateroid pterygoid	Superficial head: Infratemporal fossa Inferior head: Lateral surface of the pterygoid plate	Capsule of the temporomandibular joint The neck of the condyle	Opening the mouth Protrusion Contralateral excursion

elevation and retrusion of the mandible, and the posterior portion results in retrusion of the mandible (Table 1.1). This muscle also helps in the ipsilateral excursion of the mandible. The temporalis is innervated by the deep temporal branch of the mandibular nerve of the trigeminal nerve, and the blood is supplied by the anterior, posterior, and superficial temporal arteries [1].

1.3.2 Masseter

The masseter muscle is rectangle-shaped and it arises from the zygomatic arch and descends to the angle of the mandible and the lateral aspect of the lower border of the mandibular ramus (Figure 1.8B) [1]. It consists of two portions: the superficial portion (pass downward and a bit backward) and the deep portion (pass chiefly in a vertical direction). Elevation of the mandible happens when the fibers of the masseter muscle contract (Table 1.1). This is a strong muscle that aids in supplying the required force for efficient chewing. The superficial portion helps in the protrusion of the mandible. The masseter is innervated by the masseteric nerve from the mandibular branch of the trigeminal nerve, and the blood is supplied by the masseteric artery [1].

1.3.3 Medial Pterygoid

The medial surface (deep or internal) of the pterygoid originates from the pterygoid fossa and stretches downward, backward, and outward; it then inserts along the medial surface of the angle of the mandible (Figure 1.9A) [1]. The superficial head of the medial pterygoid

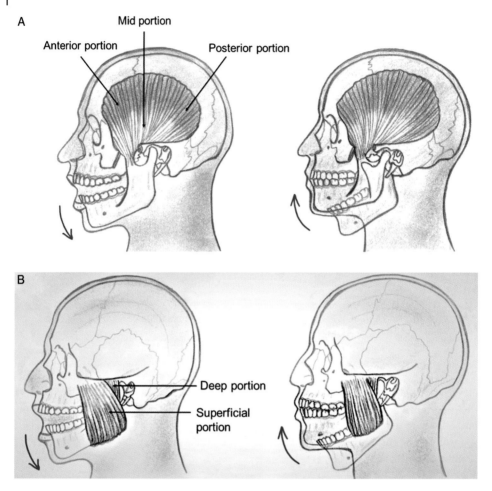

Figure 1.8 Temporalis and masseter muscle in function during opening (depression) and closing (elevation). A, Temporalis muscle in function during opening and closing of the mandible. B, Masseter muscle in function during opening and closing of the mandible. Adapted from Reference [1]; chapter published in Management of Temporomandibular Disorders and Occlusion, 7th edition, Okeson J.P., Functional Anatomy and Biomechanics of the Masticatory System, page 11, 13, Copyright Elsevier (2013).

originates from the maxillary tuberosity, runs along with the masseter muscle, and inserts at the ramus of the mandible. The medial pterygoid results in the elevation of the mandible as a result of the contractions of the muscle fibers (Table 1.1). It is effective in mandibular protrusion as well. Contralateral excursive movement is created by the unilateral contraction of this muscle. The medial is innervated by the mandibular branch of the trigeminal nerve and the blood is supplied by the pterygoid branch of the maxillary artery [1].

1.3.4 Lateral Pterygoid

The lateral pterygoid is divided into two distinct and different muscles: the inferior and superior lateral pterygoids. Their functions are quite different. The superior head of the lateral pterygoid muscle is smaller and originates from the infratemporal surface of the greater

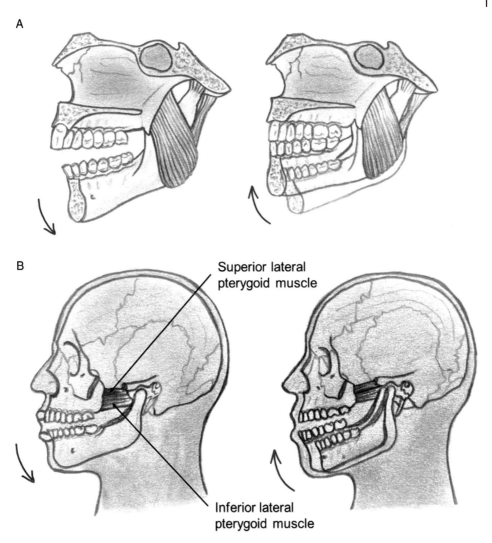

Figure 1.9 Medial, inferior, and superior lateral pterygoid muscles during opening (depression) and closing (elevation). A, Medial pterygoid in function during opening and closing of the mandible. B, Inferior and superior lateral pterygoid muscles in function during opening and closing of the mandible. Adapted from Reference [1]; chapter published in Management of Temporomandibular Disorders and Occlusion, 7th edition, Okeson J.P., Functional Anatomy and Biomechanics of the Masticatory System, page 13–14, Copyright Elsevier (2013).

wing of the sphenoid, stretching quite horizontally, backward, and outward; it then inserts in the articular capsule, the disc, and the condylar neck (Figure 1.9B) [1]. Most of its fibers, i.e. 60–70%, attach to the condylar neck, and just 30–40% attach to the disc [6, 26]. The inferior head of the lateral pterygoid emerges from the outer area of the lateral pterygoid plate and stretches upward, backward, and outward; it then inserts predominantly on the condylar neck (Figure 1.9B) [1]. As the simultaneous contraction of the left and right inferior lateral pterygoids happens, there is a forward pull of the condyles below the articular eminences, resulting in mandibular protrusion. Contralateral excursive movement is created by unilateral contraction and brings about lateral mandibular movement to the opposite side (Table 1.1). During the opening, only the inferior lateral pterygoid becomes active, while the superior lateral pterygoid only becomes active when united with the elevator muscles. It also becomes specifically active in the power stroke and during the moment when teeth are in occlusion. Power stroke indicates the motions of the mandible as opposed to resistance, for instance, chewing/clenching. The lateral pterygoid pulls the condyle and the disc, primarily in an anterior aspect. The medial angulation of the muscles' pull is enhanced when there is forward movement of the condyle. The muscle pull is directed more medially rather than anteriorly when the mouth is widely opened. The superior and inferior lateral pterygoids are innervated by the pterygoid branch of the trigeminal nerve and the blood is supplied by the pterygoid branch of the maxillary artery [1].

1.3.5 Accessory Muscles of Mastication

Accessory muscles of mastication that are directly associated with mandibular function and assist in jaw opening include the digastric, mylohyoid, geniohyoid, omohyoid, sternohyoid, stylohyoid, sternothyroid, and thyrohyoid muscles. These muscles coordinate the full integration of mandibular movement during opening and closing through their attachments to the hyoid bone, the mandible, and other bones [1, 2].

Accessory muscles that are indirectly associated with mandibular function are in the cervical area and include the sternocleidomastoid and scalenus anterior, scalenus medius, and scalenus posterior muscles. These muscles help in the stabilization of the skull and neck and allow the mandible to move relative to the skull [1, 2].

The digastric muscle is divided into two portions (Figure 1.10) [1]. The anterior belly of the digastric muscle originates at the fossa present on the mandible's lingual surface, exactly over

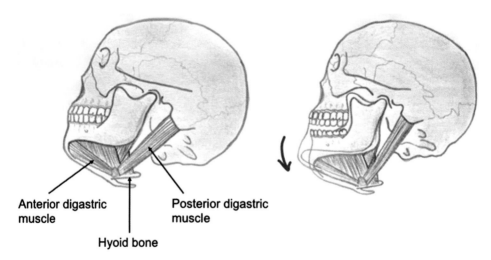

Anterior digastric muscle

Posterior digastric muscle

Hyoid bone

Figure 1.10 Digastric muscle in function during opening (depression) and closing (elevation) of the mandible. Adapted from Reference [1]; chapter published in Management of Temporomandibular Disorders and Occlusion, 7th edition, Okeson J.P., Functional Anatomy and Biomechanics of the Masticatory System, page 15, Copyright Elsevier (2013).

the lower border and near the midline, and the fibers of this muscle pass downward and backward and then insert at the very same intermediate tendon where the posterior belly of the digastric joins. The posterior belly of the digastric muscle arises from the mastoid notch and the fibers of this muscle pass forward, downward, and inward to form the intermediate tendon joined to the hyoid bone. The contraction of the left and right digastric muscles and the fixation of hyoid bone through the support of infrahyoid and suprahyoid muscles results in the lowering and backward pull of the mandible, which separates the teeth from the contact. As the mandible becomes stable, the hyoid bone is elevated by the infrahyoid and suprahyoid along with the digastric muscles, which is a crucial activity in the process of swallowing. The mandibular function is well coordinated by the infrahyoid and suprahyoid muscles. The anterior digastric is innervated by the mandibular branch of the trigeminal nerve and mylohyoid nerve, and blood is supplied by the submental artery [1]. The posterior digastric is innervated by the digastric branch of the facial nerve and the blood is supplied by the facial and lingual arteries. The strap muscles primarily function to raise and depress the hyoid bone and larynx. The strap muscles also assist with depression of the mandible when opening the mouth against an opposing force. The buccinator is a facial expression muscle that helps in mastication by keeping food pushed back within the oral cavity [27].

1.3.6   Clinical Considerations of the Muscles of Mastication

TMJ pain and dysfunction may result from various etiologies. They are commonly seen in nocturnal bruxism, habitual clenching of the mouth, and trauma to the TMJ from injury. Bruxism is a common cause of TMJ dysfunction, secondary to a resultant imbalance in the muscle of mastication forces from excessive grinding of the teeth [28, 29]. Muscle spasms of the muscles of mastication (trismus) can be a symptom of a tumor or infection, which can result in difficulty in opening the mouth. Other infections or inflammation of the muscles may present as myositis or pain during the movement of the jaw [30]. TMJ dysfunction can also result from the imbalance of forces within the muscles of mastication.

Damage or disease in the TMJ area adversely affects masticatory function. Masticatory muscle disorders include myofascial pain and dysfunction, myositis, and neoplasms. The masticator space is enveloped by the deep cervical facia; hence, tumors of TMJ are rare. The tumors of TMJ might have extended from adjacent regions. Mesially, the fascia is attached to the skull base, laterally to the temporalis muscle, anteriorly to the body of the mandible, and posteriorly to the ramus of the mandible [31].

1.4   Structures and Functions of Teeth and Associated Structures

In humans, the dentition comprises 32 permanent teeth as shown in (Figure 1.11). A tooth consists of two parts: crown and root (Figure 1.12). The part that can be seen above the gingival tissue is the crown, and the section of the tooth that is surrounded by and submerged in the alveolar bone is the root. Numerous fibers of connective tissues help in attaching the root to the alveolar bone.

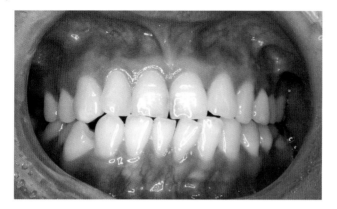

Figure 1.11 Human dentition showing upper, lower teeth, and gingiva.

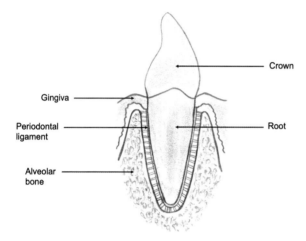

Figure 1.12 The tooth and surrounding structures.

Most of the fibers obliquely begin from the cementum and then to the bone in a cervical direction (Figure 1.12). Collectively, the fibers can be termed the periodontal ligament. In addition to firmly attaching the tooth to the bony socket, the fibers also aid in the dissipation of the forces on the bone, which are applied during the teeth's functional contact (natural shock absorber). The information related to position and pressure is provided by specialized receptors, which are a part of the periodontal ligament.

Both the maxillary and mandibular arches consist of the alveolar bone where the distribution of the 32 permanent teeth is equal – alignment of the 16 maxillary teeth is in the maxilla's alveolar process that is firmly linked to the lower anterior part of the skull; the alveolar process of the mandible, the jaw which can move, contains the alignment of the remaining 16 teeth. Usually, the mandibular teeth overlap with the maxillary teeth when in occlusion, both horizontally and vertically, mainly due to the mandibular arch being smaller than the maxillary arch. The reasons for this discrepancy in size are that (i) the mandibular teeth widths are narrower than the maxillary anterior teeth, creating a smaller arch width and (ii) the facial angulation of the mandibular anterior teeth is smaller than the maxillary anterior teeth, which ultimately results in some vertical and horizontal overlapping.

Incisors are the teeth that are situated in the arches' most anterior region. These exhibit a typical shovel shape, also consisting of an incisal edge. Both maxillary and mandibular sections consist of four incisors each. The incisors are responsible for cutting off food in the process of mastication. The canines are posterior to the incisors situated at the arches' corners. In general, they are the longest among the permanent teeth and they consist of a root and a single cusp. Both maxillary and mandibular sections consist of two canines each. As we move further back in position in the arch, we find the premolars. Both maxillary and mandibular regions each consist of four premolars. Since they have two cusps, they are also known as bicuspids. With two cusps present, the biting surfaces of premolars increase greatly. The occlusion of mandibular and maxillary premolars is such that food is caught and crushed in between the teeth. Premolars are mainly responsible for effectively breaking down the substances of food into minute sizes. Molars are the teeth found behind the premolars. Both the mandibular and maxillary sections consist of six molars each. There are either four or five cusps in the crown of each molar. Due to this, a surface that is large and broad is created, which is enough to accomplish the disintegrating and crushing of food. Molars are functionally special in the latter chewing stages. In that stage, the breakdown of food into small particles is suitable for swallowing.

1.5 Biomechanical Interaction Between Masticatory Muscles and Bones

Mechanical stimulation in the orofacial region is an important factor in the determination of bone shape and its development. The mechanical stimulation results in bone strains above the 1500–3000 microstrain range, and the strain results in bone modeling, which increases bone mass [32, 33]. On the other hand, strains below the 100–300 microstrain activate bone resorption and this reduces unnecessary bone. In addition, low strain magnitudes acting at high frequency also result in bone formation [34, 35]. For bone formation to occur, bone cells that are responsible for bone remodeling must sense such changes in mechanical stimuli. During muscle contraction and functional loading, i.e. the deformation of bone tissue, intertrabecular spaces, and movement of interstitial fluids cause mechanical stimuli that osteocytes sense through mechanoreceptors to activate the target molecule within the cell [20].

The masticatory apparatus produces loads of different magnitudes and high frequencies on the jaws and teeth. These loads result in bone remodeling and ultimately shape the mandible to fit mechanically. These loads result in micro deformation because of the different force vectors acting on it.

During the chewing stroke and muscle activity, bone strain occurs and the TMJ acts as the fulcrum; the distance of muscle insertion to the TMJ is the force arm, and the biting force is the resistance arm. The more anterior the biting point, the lower the resulting biting force, and vice versa. As the posterior teeth are close to the TMJ, biting at the posterior teeth reduces the length of the resistance arm and increases bite force. Hence, biting in posterior teeth is more efficient in terms of the use of muscle force. There is also a difference in the TMJ loading vectors for molar and premolar bites due to the bite-point location [36]. The posterior part of the mandible has a thinner cortical bone compared to the anterior part of the mandible, which can absorb the strains during biting [37, 38].

Furthermore, during biting, the TMJ surfaces apart from the forces on the mandible and cranium [36, 39]. The muscle force decomposes at the biting point and the TMJ. Thus, if a large force is generated during contraction, it reduces the reaction force at the TMJ. The resulting forces produced during biting cause the deformation of the mandible in three patterns: bending of the sagittal plane, bending of the transverse plane, and twisting of the body and symphysis [40, 41] as shown in Figure 1.13 [20]. The anterior part of the mandible has a thick cortical bone, and the posterior end of the corpus has more strains during biting [37, 38].

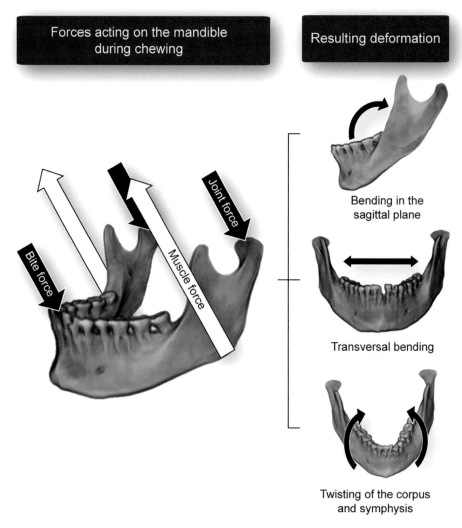

Figure 1.13 Various forces acting on the mandible during biting and bone deformation. Reference [20] / Frontiers Media S.A. / CC BY 4.0.

References

1 Okeson, J.P., *Management of Temporomandibular Disorders and Occlusion*. 7th ed. 2013, St. Louis, Missouri: Mosby.

2 Dawson, P.E., *Functional Occlusion From TMJ to Smile Design*. 2007, St. Louis: CV Mosby.

3 Sava, A. and M.M. Scutariu, Functional anatomy of the temporomandibular joint (I). *Rev Med Chir Soc Med Nat Iasi*, 2012. **116**(3): p. 902–906.

4 Sava, A. and M.M. Scutariu, Functional anatomy of the temporo-mandibular joint (II). *Rev Med Chir Soc Med Nat Iasi*, 2012. **116**(4): p. 1213–1217.

5 Acri, T.M., K. Shin, D. Seol, N.Z. Laird, I. Song, S.M. Geary, J.L. Chakka, J.A. Martin, and A.K. Salem, Tissue engineering for the temporomandibular joint. *Adv Healthc Mater*, 2019. **8**(2): p. e1801236.

6 Carpentier, P., J.P. Yung, R. Marguelles-Bonnet, and M. Meunissier, Insertions of the lateral pterygoid muscle: an anatomic study of the human temporomandibular joint. *J Oral Maxillofac Surg*, 1988. **46**(6): p. 477–482.

7 Fernandes, P.R., H.A. de Vasconsellos, J.P. Okeson, R.L. Bastos, and M.L. Maia, The anatomical relationship between the position of the auriculotemporal nerve and mandibular condyle. *Cranio*, 2003. **21**(3): p. 165–171.

8 Cuccia, A.M., C. Caradonna, D. Caradonna, G. Anastasi, D. Milardi, A. Favaloro, A. De Pietro, T.M. Angileri, L. Caradonna, and G. Cutroneo, The arterial blood supply of the temporomandibular joint: an anatomical study and clinical implications. *Imaging Sci Dent*, 2013. **43**(1): p. 37–44.

9 Helland, M.M., Anatomy and function of the temporomandibular joint. *J Orthop Sports Phys Ther*, 1980. **1**(3): p. 145–152.

10 Shaffer, S.M., J.M. Brismée, P.S. Sizer, and C.A. Courtney, Temporomandibular disorders. Part 1: anatomy and examination/diagnosis. *J Man Manip Ther*, 2014. **22**(1): p. 2–12.

11 Jung, H.D., S.Y. Kim, H.S. Park, and Y.S. Jung, Orthognathic surgery and temporomandibular joint symptoms. *Maxillofac Plast Reconstr Surg*, 2015. **37**(1): p. 14.

12 Talmaceanu, D., L.M. Lenghel, N. Bolog, M. Hedesiu, S. Buduru, H. Rotar, M. Baciut, and G. Baciut, Imaging modalities for temporomandibular joint disorders: an update. *Clujul Med*, 2018. **91**(3): p. 280–287.

13 Brooks, S.L., J.W. Brand, S.J. Gibbs, L. Hollender, A.G. Lurie, K.A. Omnell, P.L. Westesson, and S.C. White, Imaging of the temporomandibular joint: a position paper of the American Academy of Oral and Maxillofacial Radiology. *Oral Surg Oral Med Oral Pathol Oral Radiol Endod*, 1997. **83**(5): p. 609–618.

14 Tsiklakis, K., K. Syriopoulos, and H.C. Stamatakis, Radiographic examination of the temporomandibular joint using cone beam computed tomography. *Dentomaxillofac Radiol*, 2004. **33**(3): p. 196–201.

15 Christensen, L.V. and G.J. Ziebert, Effects of experimental loss of teeth on the temporomandibular joint. *J Oral Rehabil*, 1986. **13**(6): p. 587–598.

16 Rokaya, D., K. Suttagul, S. Joshi, B.P. Bhattarai, P.K. Shah, and S. Dixit, An epidemiological study on the prevalence of temporomandibular disorder and associated history and problems in Nepalese subjects. *J Dent Anesth Pain Med*, 2018. **18**(1): p. 27–33.

17 Murakami, K., N. Segami, M. Okamoto, I. Yamamura, K. Takahashi, and Y. Tsuboi, Outcome of arthroscopic surgery for internal derangement of the temporomandibular joint: long-term results covering 10 years. *J Craniomaxillofac Surg*, 2000. **28**(5): p. 264–271.

18 Tzanidakis, K. and A.J. Sidebottom, Outcomes of open temporomandibular joint surgery following failure to improve after arthroscopy: is there an algorithm for success? *Br J Oral Maxillofac Surg*, 2013. **51**(8): p. 818–821.

19 Sciote, J.J., M.J. Horton, A.M. Rowlerson, and J. Link, Specialized cranial muscles: how different are they from limb and abdominal muscles? *Cells Tissues Organs*, 2003. **174**(1–2): p. 73–86.

20 Buvinic, S., J. Balanta-Melo, K. Kupczik, W. Vásquez, C. Beato, and V. Toro-Ibacache, Muscle-bone crosstalk in the masticatory system: from biomechanical to molecular interactions. *Front Endocrinol (Lausanne)*, 2020. **11**: p. 606947.

21 Isola, G., G.P. Anastasi, G. Matarese, R.C. Williams, G. Cutroneo, P. Bracco, and M.G. Piancino, Functional and molecular outcomes of the human masticatory muscles. *Oral Dis*, 2018. **24**(8): p. 1428–1441.

22 Akintoye, S.O., T. Lam, S. Shi, J. Brahim, M.T. Collins, and P.G. Robey, Skeletal site-specific characterization of orofacial and iliac crest human bone marrow stromal cells in same individuals. *Bone*, 2006. **38**(6): p. 758–768.

23 Akintoye, S.O., The distinctive jaw and alveolar bone regeneration. *Oral Dis*, 2018. **24**(1–2): p. 49–51.

24 Singhal, V., L.P. Torre Flores, F.C. Stanford, A.T. Toth, B. Carmine, M. Misra, and M.A. Bredella, Differential associations between appendicular and axial marrow adipose tissue with bone microarchitecture in adolescents and young adults with obesity. *Bone*, 2018. **116**: p. 203–206.

25 Li, C., F. Wang, R. Zhang, P. Qiao, and H. Liu, Comparison of proliferation and osteogenic differentiation potential of rat mandibular and femoral bone marrow mesenchymal stem cells in vitro. *Stem Cells Dev*, 2020. **29**(11): p. 728–736.

26 Dusek, T.O. and J.P. Kiely, Quantifcation of the superior lateral pterygoid insertion on TMJ components. *J Dent Res*, 1991. **70**: p. 421.

27 Alomar, X., J. Medrano, J. Cabratosa, J.A. Clavero, M. Lorente, I. Serra, J.M. Monill, and A. Salvador, Anatomy of the temporomandibular joint. *Semin Ultrasound CT MR*, 2007. **28**(3): p. 170–183.

28 Finden, S.G., W.S. Enochs, and V.M. Rao, Pathologic changes of the lateral pterygoid muscle in patients with derangement of the temporomandibular joint disk: objective measures at MR imaging. *AJNR Am J Neuroradiol*, 2007. **28**(8): p. 1537–1539.

29 Taneja, P., R. Nagpal, C.M. Marya, S. Kataria, V. Sahay, and D. Goyal, Temporomandibular disorders among adolescents of Haryana, India: a cross-sectional study. *Int J Clin Pediatr Dent*, 2019. **12**(6): p. 500–506.

30 Karlsson, O., T. Karlsson, N. Pauli, P. Andréll, and C. Finizia, Jaw exercise therapy for the treatment of trismus in head and neck Cancer: a prospective three-year follow-up study. *Support Care Cancer*, 2021. **29**(7): p. 3793–3800.

31 Chughtai, S., K.A. Chughtai, S. Montoya, and A.A. Bhatt, Radiographic review of anatomy and pathology of the masticator space: what the emergency radiologist needs to know. *Emerg Radiol*, 2020. **27**(3): p. 329–339.

32 Frost, H.M., Bone's mechanostat: a 2003 update. *Anat Rec A Discov Mol Cell Evol Biol*, 2003. **275**(2): p. 1081–1101.

33 Frost, H.M., Bone "mass" and the "mechanostat": a proposal. *Anat Rec*, 1987. **219**(1): p. 1–9.

34 Lad, S.E., W.S. McGraw, and D.J. Daegling, Haversian remodeling corresponds to load frequency but not strain magnitude in the macaque (Macaca fascicularis) skeleton. *Bone*, 2019. **127**: p. 571–576.

35 Hsieh, Y.F. and C.H. Turner, Effects of loading frequency on mechanically induced bone formation. *J Bone Miner Res*, 2001. **16**(5): p. 918–924.

36 Abe, M., R.U. Medina-Martinez, K. Itoh, and S. Kohno, Temporomandibular joint loading generated during bilateral static bites at molars and premolars. *Med Biol Eng Comput*, 2006. **44**(11): p. 1017–1030.

37 Daegling, D.J., The relationship of in vivo bone strain to mandibular corpus morphology in Macaca fascicularis. *J Hum Evol*, 1993. **25**(4): p. 247–269.

38 Fukase, H., Functional significance of bone distribution in the human mandibular symphysis. *Anthropol Sci*, 2007. **115**: p. 55–62.

39 Naeije, M. and N. Hofman, Biomechanics of the human temporomandibular joint during chewing. *J Dent Res*, 2003. **82**(7): p. 528–531.

40 Hylander, W.L., Stress and strain in the mandibular symphysis of primates: a test of competing hypotheses. *Am J Phys Anthropol*, 1984. **64**(1): p. 1–46.

41 Gröning, F., J. Liu, M.J. Fagan, and P. O'Higgins, Why do humans have chins? Testing the mechanical significance of modern human symphyseal morphology with finite element analysis. *Am J Phys Anthropol*, 2011. **144**(4): p. 593–606.

2

Intra-arch Tooth Alignment

2.1 Introduction

Inter-arch tooth alignment can be described as the interrelation of the teeth present in one arch to the teeth present in the other arch. Like in the closure of the mandible, when there is contact between the two arches, the establishment of the teeth's occlusal relationship takes place.

2.2 Maxillary and Mandibular Arch

The teeth are arranged in crescent-shaped dental arches in the maxilla and mandible. Each jaw consists of an arch (maxilla and mandible), constituting the dentition together (Figure 2.1). The dimensions of the dental arch, including length, width, and form, are vital for the diagnosis, treatment planning, and treatment, as well as the outcome of the treatment. These factors are concerned with patients of all age groups seeking orthodontic treatment.

2.2.1 Arch Form

The shape of the dental arch in the maxillary or mandibular is known as the arch form (Figure 2.2). Chuck [2] first classified the dental arch into three different forms: ovoid, tapered, and square shapes. There can be different combinations, such as ovoid, narrow ovoid, tapered, and narrow tapered [1].

The arch is a key determinant in teeth position and the teeth selection, and position is based on the functional and esthetic needs of the patient [3–6]. It was found that there is a correlation between arch form and facial form. It was found that 63.63% of individuals with the long faces (leptoprosopic) had squarish arch forms, while 54.6% with average faces (mesoprosopic) had ovoid arch forms [3].

Morphological differences exist among various ethnic backgrounds and populations. The ovoid arch form was the most common among the Egyptian population, followed by the square arch form, while the tapered arch form was the least common one [7]. Similarly, in the Jordanian population, the ovoid (catenary) arch form was the most prevalent, followed

Introduction to the Masticatory System and Dental Occlusion, First Edition. Dinesh Rokaya.
© 2025 John Wiley & Sons Ltd. Published 2025 by John Wiley & Sons Ltd.

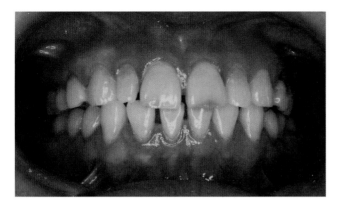

Figure 2.1 Maxillary arch and mandibular arch.

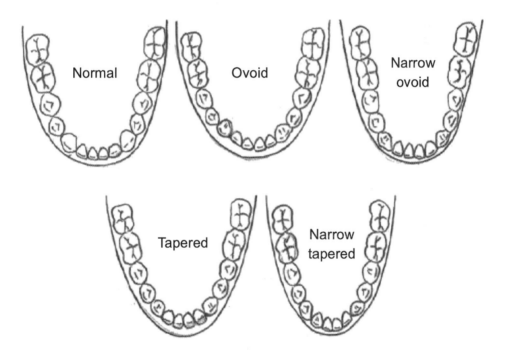

Figure 2.2 Types of arch forms. Adapted from Reference [1].

by the wide elliptical form [4]. The other forms, tudor (ovoid tapering), tapered equilateral, and quadrangular forms, were less frequent. Regarding size, medium size was the most prevalent among the studied samples. On the contrary, Nojima et al. [8] found that there is no single arch form specific to any of the angle classifications or ethnic groups (Caucasian and Japanese), and the frequency of a particular arch form varies among angle classifications or ethnic groups. They also found that no significant difference in arch dimensions was observed between the two ethnic groups. The Caucasians showed significantly increased arch depth and decreased arch width compared with the Japanese population.

2.2.2 Arch Length

It can be defined as the interspace between the distal surface of the third molar on one side and the distal surface of the third molar on the opposite side of the jaw. It is passed through proximal contact at all positions.

Significant changes in the maxillary and mandibular arch length relationship occur after the eruption of the deciduous dentition (approximately four years) till the eruption of the second molars (approximately 13.3 years) [9–11]. Bishara et al. [9] did a longitudinal study on the changes in maxillary and mandibular arch length over a 45-year period. They found that the greatest incremental increases occurred during the first two years of life. Arch length continued to increase until 13 years in the maxillary arch and until eight years in the mandibular arch. Then, a significant and consistent decrease occurred in both maxillary and mandibular arches, mesial to the permanent first molars.

2.2.3 Arch Width

It is the distance between the canines, bicuspids, and the first molars in the maxillary or mandibular arch (Figure 2.3). These distances establish the shape and size of the dental arch. The males have larger maxillary and mandibular dental arch width and dental arch depth compared to the females [12].

Like the arch length, changes in the maxillary and mandibular arch width relationship occur after the eruption of the deciduous dentition till the eruption of the second molars. Bishara et al. [9] did a longitudinal study on the changes in intercanine and intermolar widths over a 45-year span and did the following: (i) Before the complete eruption of the deciduous dentition (six weeks and two years old), there is a significant increase in the maxillary and mandibular anterior and posterior arch widths. (ii) Intercanine and intermolar widths significantly increased between 3 and 13 years old in both the maxillary and mandibular arches, and following the complete eruption of the permanent dentition,

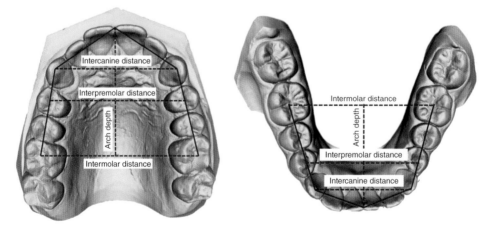

Figure 2.3 Various arch widths in the maxillary and mandibular arch. Reference [12] / Springer Nature / CC BY 4.0.

there is a slight decrease in the dental arch widths, more in the intercanine than in the intermolar widths. (iii) After the eruption of the four incisors, mandibular intercanine width is established by eight years old. After the eruption of the permanent dentition, there is either no or only a slight decrease in arch widths.

Harris [13] did a study on the changes in arch size and shape at about 20 years of age and again at about 55 years. He found that the arch width increased over time, especially in the distal segments, whereas the arch length decreased. These changes significantly altered the shape of the arch toward shorter, broader arches. The data suggest that changes during adulthood occur most rapidly during the second and third decades of life, but do not stop thereafter.

2.2.4 Arch Circumference

The extent between the distal surface of the second primary molar (in other words, the permanent first molar's mesial surface) of one arch side to the same surface on the opposite arch is known as the arch circumference.

Dental arch perimeter, including length and width, is considered to be important for diagnosis and treatment, especially in orthodontics [14]. The arch circumference can be measured conventionally, digitally (3D virtually), or using an equation [14–16]. The conventional method shows better overall reproducibility compared to the 3D virtual method [15]. Still, the measurements with digital models are comparable to those derived from plaster models [16], and reproducibility obtained from the 3D virtual method is also acceptable for clinical use [15].

2.3 Planes of Occlusion

The plane of occlusion consists of three curves: the curve of Wilson, the curve of Spee, and the curve of Monsoon.

2.3.1 Curve of Spee

It is a continuous line that passes through the buccal cusps of posterior teeth, which is convex in the maxilla and concave in the mandible [17]. This curvature is seen from the lateral view (Figure 2.4) [18]. On average, the curvature of the arc is a part of a circle with a four-inch radius. The development of the curve of Spee results from a combination of factors, including an eruption of teeth (primary, mixed, and permanent dentition), growth of orofacial structures, and development of the neuromuscular system [19, 20]. It has been found that the mandibular sagittal and vertical position relative to the cranium is related to the curve of Spee [21]. The curve of Spee is increased in brachycephalic (short) facial form and short mandible [22, 23]. The presence of a curve of Spee makes it possible for a dentition to resist the occlusion forces during mastication [20, 24]. It has been found that the curve of Spee in the deciduous dentition ranges from flat to mild, whereas in adults, it is more pronounced [24, 25]. It shows the greatest depth in the early mixed dentition because of the eruption of the permanent first molar and central incisor; the depth reaches a maximum with the eruption of the permanent second

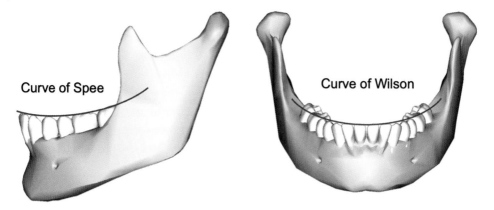

Curve of Spee

Curve of Wilson

Figure 2.4 Curves of occlusion: the curve of Spee and the curve of Wilson. Adapted and modified from Reference [18].

molars and then remains stable after late adolescence and early adulthood. Once established, the curve of Spee is relatively stable throughout life [26, 27]. The curve of Spee in Class II malocclusions shows a deeper pattern than in other malocclusions [28].

An exaggerated curve of Spee is commonly found in dental malocclusions in patients with a deep bite [24]. An excessive curve of Spee alters the muscle imbalance and leads to improper functional occlusion [29]. The goal of orthodontic treatment should focus on flattening the occlusal plane, especially in patients with deep bite [30–32]. Correction of the exaggerated curve of Spee can be done by the intrusion of incisors and/or extrusion of molars [24].

2.3.2 Curve of Wilson

It is a line that passes through the lingual and buccal cusps of the posterior teeth on both the left and right jaws [17]. It is seen from the frontal view (Figure 2.4) [18, 33]. The variability in the curves of occlusion (curve of Spee and Wilson) comes from genetic differences with little contribution from environmental factors [34]. The siblings show mostly similar occlusal curves.

2.3.3 Sphere of Monsoon

It consists of two curves: the curve of Spee and the Curve of Wilson on the occlusal surface of the teeth. It is viewed in 3D as a pyramid with a radius of four inches and a curved base that resembles part of a sphere (Figure 2.5) [33].

2.4 Buccolingual Occlusal Contact Relationship

While the dental arches are seen from the occlusal aspect, particular landmarks that clarify the interocclusal relationship of the teeth can be envisioned.

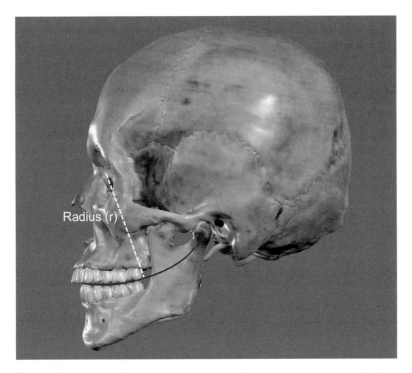

Figure 2.5 Curves of Spee showing the radius (r). Image taken from the Anatomage Table (Anatomage Inc., California, USA).

2.4.1 Bucco-occlusal Line

The B-O is an imaginary line that passes through the buccal cusp tips of all the posterior teeth of the mandible. In a typical arch, the B-O line courses in a continuous and smooth manner, giving out the general arch form. Also, this line presents a division between the outer and inner sides of the buccal cusps.

2.4.2 Linguo-occlusal Line

The L-O is an imaginary line passing through the lingual cusps of all the posterior teeth of the maxilla. In a regular arch form, the L-O line presents a division between the inner and outer sides of these centric cusps (Figure 2.6) [17].

2.4.3 Central Fossa Line

The C-F line is an imaginary line passing through the central developmental grooves of posterior teeth of the mandible and maxilla. In general, well-aligned arch, the C-F line is uninterrupted and discloses the arch form. The C-F line of maxillary teeth occludes with the B-O line of mandibular teeth. Concurrently, the C-F line of mandibular teeth occludes with the L-O line of maxillary teeth.

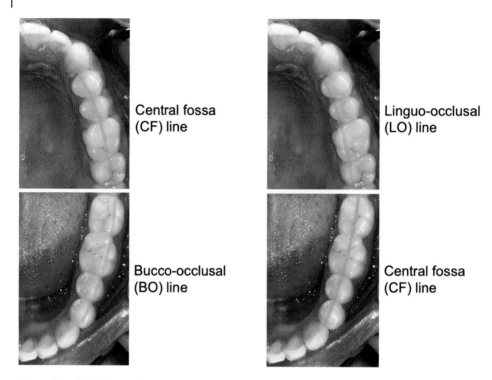

Central fossa
(CF) line

Linguo-occlusal
(LO) line

Bucco-occlusal
(BO) line

Central fossa
(CF) line

Figure 2.6 Maxillary and mandibular arch showing the central fossa (C-F) line, bucco-occlusal (B-O) line, and linguo-occlusal (L-O) line.

Following the drawing of the C-F line, proximal contact areas can be located, which are usually detected as somewhat buccal to the central fossa line (Figure 2.6) [17]. This permits a large area of lingual embrasures and a small area of buccal embrasures. The greater lingual embrasures function as a major spillway for food bolus during mastication.

2.5 Mesio-Distal Relationship and Buccolingual Embrasure

In the condition where the centric cusps contact the opposite central fossa line, occlusal contact takes place. The centric cusps basically contact in one of the two areas from the facial aspect: (i) C-F line and (ii) marginal ridge and embrasure areas (Figure 2.7) [17]. According to the Glossary of Prosthodontic Terms 9 (GPT-9), the embrasures are the spaces defined by the surfaces of two adjacent teeth [35]. There are four embrasure spaces in each proximal contact area: incisal/occlusal, mesial, distal, and gingival embrasure.

When two unlike curved surfaces of C-F areas connect, just specific parts unite at a particular time, withdrawing other areas free from contact and acting as spillways for the food being crushed. When there is a mandibular shift during the process of mastication, various contact areas are created, resulting in several spillways. This shift of mandible magnifies masticatory efficiency.

Figure 2.7 The proximal contact areas, buccal embrasure, lingual embrasure, and C-F line in posterior teeth (maxillary teeth).

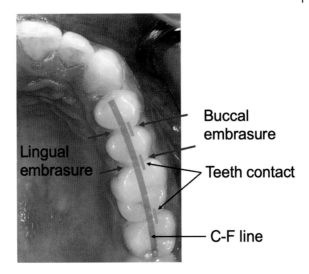

Buccal embrasure

Lingual embrasure

Teeth contact

C-F line

Another form of occlusal contact is between marginal ridges and cusp tips. Faintly raised areas that are convex, situated at the mesial and distal edges of occlusal surfaces, which connect with the interproximal teeth surfaces, are known as marginal ridges. The part of the marginal ridge that is mostly elevated is moderately convex. So, the contact type is well represented by the cusp tip that contacts a flat surface. In this correlation, the cusp tip smoothly penetrates along the food, and spillways are allowed in every direction.

As the regular inter-arch tooth relation is seen from the lateral view, it is observed that each tooth occludes two opposite teeth. The indicated relation aids in distributing occlusal forces to many teeth and, eventually, to the whole arch. In addition, it assists in maintaining arch integrity to some level, even in a condition where there is tooth loss, as balancing occlusal contacts are yet sustained on all existing teeth.

2.6   Proximal (Interproximal) and Occlusal Contacts

Proximal contact is the area of a tooth that is in close contact with an adjacent tooth in the same arch (GPT-9) [35] (Figure 2.8). Occlusal contact is touching opposing teeth on an elevation of the mandible (Figure 2.8). The close contact of teeth with opposing teeth in the dental arch in their maximum intercuspation is known as the maximum intercuspal position or intercuspal position (ICP). When the mandible shifts laterally from this position, noncentric contact will occur and guide it. Moreover, noncentric cusps complete the guiding contacts that control chewing stroke during mastication. Hence, these cusps are also correctly mentioned as guiding cusps.

2.7   Functional Form of the Teeth at their Incisal and Occlusal Thirds

Teeth form is harmonious with the function they carry out and their position and arrangement in structures concerned with oral motor behavior, particularly mastication (Figure 2.9).

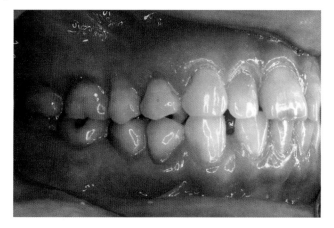

Figure 2.8 Proximal contacts in maxillary and mandibular teeth.

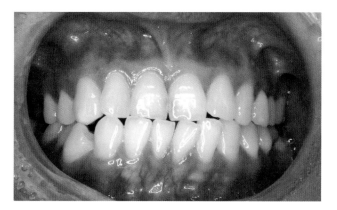

Figure 2.9 Teeth form and their position and arrangement in structures.

Concave and convex surfaces are present on the incisal/occlusal third of the crown portion of teeth on all occlusal contact areas [17]. Throughout several movements of the mandible, the curved surfaces of maxillary teeth come in contact with the curved surfaces of mandibular teeth. The curved surfaces may either be concave or convex. The convex surface that presents a part of the occlusal third of a tooth might come in contact with the concave or convex part of the other tooth (Figure 2.8). The convex parts of the incisal ridges of mandibular incisors contact the concave portions of the lingual surfaces of maxillary incisors.

Even though the teeth appear to occlude relatively closer during centric occlusion, it has been known that escapements are provided. These escapement spaces are essential for an efficient occlusion in the process of mastication. In situations where there is a close approximation of occluding surfaces, few of the escapement spaces are so slight that even light is barely emitted through them. They differ in degree of opening, ranging from small to abundant, measuring a few millimeters or more at the widest part of the embrasure. In teeth that are not worn, the rounded surfaces do not engage closely with each other. Some of the features that provide escapement space in the teeth are cusps and ridges, developmental grooves and sulci, and embrasures or interdental spaces when the teeth are in occlusion.

2.8   Inclination and Angulations of Individual Teeth

When the dental arches are observed from a lateral view, the mesiodistal axial relation can be noticed. When the lines are drawn out along the long axes of the roots, occlusal from the crowns, the teeth angulation with regard to the alveolar bone can be viewed. In the case of the maxillary arch, anterior as well as posterior teeth are inclined mesially, and the second and third molars are inclined to a greater extent than the premolars [17, 36]. In the case of the mandibular arch, a distinct form of inclination is seen as shown in Figure 2.10 [18].

Similarly, when the dental arches are seen from the frontal view, the buccolingual axial relation can be observed. Normally, the posterior teeth of the maxillary arch have a slight buccal inclination (Figure 2.10) [18], while the mandibular posterior teeth have a slight lingual inclination [17, 36]. Racial and ethnic factors contribute to variations in crown angulations and crown inclinations [37].

The teeth are set up with proper angulation and inclination in complete denture treatment (Figure 2.11) [38–41]. In addition, teeth angulation and inclination are important in orthodontics in teeth alignment [42]. Proper relationships, such as the mesio-distal width

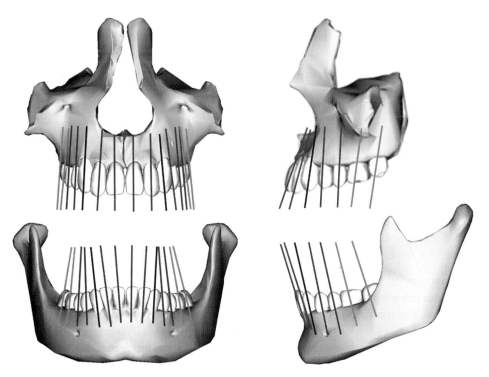

Figure 2.10   Maxillary and mandibular teeth angulation on the frontal and lateral view. Adapted and modified from Reference [18].

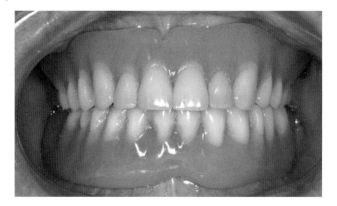

Figure 2.11 Ideal teeth alignment in artificial teeth in the maxillary and mandibular complete denture.

of the maxillary dentition and the mesio-distal width of the mandibular dentition, including the angulation and inclination, will favor an optimal post-treatment occlusion [37, 43]. An important objective of orthodontic treatment is to obtain the correct mesiodistal angulation and faciolingual inclination for all teeth. There are various methods to measure the mesiodistal angulation and faciolingual inclination for all teeth, including one-beam computed tomography [44]. The height and width of a tooth crown can either diminish or enhance the effect of angulation on the arch length [44–47].

Verma et al. [48] found that there is a highly significant correlation between teeth angulation and inclination in the maxillary and mandibular arches. The bases of different brackets adapt differently on each tooth surface and may be the source of errors in torque expression. Though the error in the expression of torque was not significant, it showed a large range, indicating the need to vary the position of brackets in different bracket systems to achieve optimum torque.

References

1 Omar, H., M. Alhajrasi, N. Felemban, and A. Hassan, Dental arch dimensions, form and tooth size ratio among a Saudi sample. *Saudi Med J*, 2018. **39**(1): p. 86–91.

2 Chuck, G.C., Ideal arch form. *Angle Orthod*, 1934. **4**(4): p. 312–327.

3 Nayar, S., S. Aruna, and W. Manzoor, Correlation between arch form and facial form: a cross sectional study. *J Pharm Bioallied Sci*, 2015. **7**(Suppl 1): p. S85–S86.

4 Aljayousi, M., S. Al-Khateeb, S. Badran, and E.S.A. Alhaija, Maxillary and mandibular dental arch forms in a Jordanian population with normal occlusion. *BMC Oral Health*, 2021. **21**(1): p. 105.

5 Balaji, S.S. and V. Bhat, A comprehensive review on the errors that occur during ideal teeth arrangement for complete denture prosthesis. *J Contemp Dent Pract*, 2018. **19**(5): p. 624–627.

6 McCord, J.F., Contemporary techniques for denture fabrication. *J Prosthodont*, 2009. **18**(2): p. 106–111.

7 Sharaf, R.F., E. Radwan, G.A. Salem, and M. Abou El-yazeed, Dental arch form and arch dimensions among a group of Egyptian children and adolescents. *Bull Natl Res Cent*, 2022. **46**(1): p. 201.

8 Nojima, K., R.P. McLaughlin, Y. Isshiki, and P.M. Sinclair, A comparative study of Caucasian and Japanese mandibular clinical arch forms. *Angle Orthod*, 2001. **71**(3): p. 195–200.

9 Bishara, S.E., J.R. Jakobsen, J. Treder, and A. Nowak, Arch length changes from 6 weeks to 45 years. *Angle Orthod*, 1998. **68**(1): p. 69–74.

10 Bishara, S.E., P. Khadivi, and J.R. Jakobsen, Changes in tooth size-arch length relationships from the deciduous to the permanent dentition: a longitudinal study. *Am J Orthod Dentofacial Orthop*, 1995. **108**(6): p. 607–613.

11 Bishara, S.E. and J.R. Jakobsen, Individual variation in tooth-size/arch-length changes from the primary to permanent dentitions. *World J Orthod*, 2006. **7**(2): p. 145–153.

12 Oliva, B., S. Sferra, A.L. Greco, F. Valente, and C. Grippaudo, Three-dimensional analysis of dental arch forms in Italian population. *Prog Orthod*, 2018. **19**(1): p. 34.

13 Harris, E.F., A longitudinal study of arch size and form in untreated adults. *Am J Orthod Dentofacial Orthop*, 1997. **111**(4): p. 419–427.

14 Al-Ansari, N.B., S.A. Abdul Ameer, and M. Nahidh, A new method for prediction of dental arch perimeter. *Clin Cosmet Investig Dent*, 2019. **11**: p. 393–397.

15 Sjögren, A.P., J.E. Lindgren, and J.A. Huggare, Orthodontic study cast analysis— reproducibility of recordings and agreement between conventional and 3D virtual measurements. *J Digit Imaging*, 2010. **23**(4): p. 482–492.

16 Fleming, P.S., V. Marinho, and A. Johal, Orthodontic measurements on digital study models compared with plaster models: a systematic review. *Orthod Craniofac Res*, 2011. **14**(1): p. 1–16.

17 Okeson, J.P., *Management of Temporomandibular Disorders and Occlusion*. 7th ed. 2013, St. Louis, Missouri: Mosby.

18 *Wikimedia Commons. Mandible close-up lateral.* https://commons.wikimedia.org *(Accessed on November 23, 2023)*. 2023.

19 da Silva, L.P. and R. Gleiser, Occlusal development between primary and mixed dentitions: a 5-year longitudinal study. *J Dent Child (Chic)*, 2008. **75**(3): p. 287–294.

20 Osborn, J.W., Orientation of the masseter muscle and the curve of Spee in relation to crushing forces on the molar teeth of primates. *Am J Phys Anthropol*, 1993. **92**(1): p. 99–106.

21 Marshall, S.D., M. Caspersen, R.R. Hardinger, R.G. Franciscus, S.A. Aquilino, and T.E. Southard, Development of the curve of Spee. *Am J Orthod Dentofacial Orthop*, 2008. **134**(3): p. 344–352.

22 Salem, O.H., F. Al-Sehaibany, and C.B. Preston, Aspects of mandibular morphology, with specific reference to the antegonial notch and the curve of Spee. *J Clin Pediatr Dent*, 2003. **27**(3): p. 261–265.

23 Wylie, W.L., Overbite and vertical facial dimensions in terms of muscle balance. *Angle Orthod*, 1994. **19**: p. 13–17.

24 Kumar, K.P. and S. Tamizharasi, Significance of curve of Spee: an orthodontic review. *J Pharm Bioallied Sci*, 2012. **4**(Suppl 2): p. S323–S328.

25 Ash Jr., M.M. and S.J. Nelson, *Wheeler's Dental Anatomy, Physiology, and Occlusion*. 8th ed. 2003, Amsterdam: Elsevier Science.

26 Bishara, S.E., J.R. Jakobsen, J.E. Treder, and M.J. Stasi, Changes in the maxillary and mandibular tooth size-arch length relationship from early adolescence to early adulthood. A longitudinal study. *Am J Orthod Dentofacial Orthop*, 1989. **95**(1): p. 46–59.

27 Carter, G.A. and J.A. McNamara, Jr., Longitudinal dental arch changes in adults. *Am J Orthod Dentofacial Orthop*, 1998. **114**(1): p. 88–99.

28 Fidler, B.C., J. Artun, D.R. Joondeph, and R.M. Little, Long-term stability of Angle Class II, division 1 malocclusions with successful occlusal results at end of active treatment. *Am J Orthod Dentofacial Orthop*, 1995. **107**(3): p. 276–285.

29 Arhakis, A. and E. Boutiou, Etiology, diagnosis, consequences and treatment of infraoccluded primary molars. *Open Dent J*, 2016. **10**: p. 714–719.

30 Garcia, R., Leveling the curve of Spee: a new prediction formula. *J Charles H Tweed Int Found*, 1985. **13**: p. 65–72.

31 Koyama, T., A comparative analysis of the curve of Spee (lateral aspect) before and after orthodontic treatment—with particular reference to overbite patients. *J Nihon Univ Sch Dent*, 1979. **21**(1–4): p. 25–34.

32 De Praeter, J., L. Dermaut, G. Martens, and A.M. Kuijpers-Jagtman, Long-term stability of the leveling of the curve of Spee. *Am J Orthod Dentofacial Orthop*, 2002. **121**(3): p. 266–272.

33 Marshall, S.D., K. Kruger, R.G. Franciscus, and T.E. Southard, Development of the mandibular curve of spee and maxillary compensating curve: a finite element model. *PLoS One*, 2019. **14**(12): p. e0221137.

34 Al-Qawasmi, R. and C. Coe, Genetic influence on the curves of occlusion in children seeking orthodontic treatment. *Int Orthod*, 2021. **19**(1): p. 82–87.

35 The glossary of prosthodontic terms: ninth edition. *J Prosthet Dent*, 2017. **117**: p. e1–e105.

36 Dempster, W.T., W.J. Adams, and R.A. Duddles, Arrangement in the jaws of the roots of the teeth. *J Am Dent Assoc*, 1963. **67**: p. 779–797.

37 Doodamani, G.M., A.S. Khala, M. Manohar, and Umashankar, Assessment of crown angulations, crown inclinations, and tooth size discrepancies in a South Indian population. *Contemp Clin Dent*, 2011. **2**(3): p. 176–181.

38 Rangarajan, V., B. Gajapathi, P.B. Yogesh, M.M. Ibrahim, R.G. Kumar, and P. Karthik, Concepts of occlusion in prosthodontics: a literature review, part I. *J Indian Prosthodont Soc*, 2015. **15**(3): p. 200–205.

39 Lang, B.R., Complete denture occlusion. *Dent Clin N Am*, 2004. **48**(3): p. 641–665, vi.

40 Beck, H.O., Occlusion as related to complete removable prosthodontics. *J Prosthet Dent*, 1972. **27**(3): p. 246–262.

41 Gibbs, C.H., P.E. Mahan, H.C. Lundeen, K. Brehnan, E.K. Walsh, and W.B. Holbrook, Occlusal forces during chewing and swallowing as measured by sound transmission. *J Prosthet Dent*, 1981. **46**(4): p. 443–449.

42 Hussels, W. and R.S. Nanda, Effect of maxillary incisor angulation and inclination on arch length. *Am J Orthod Dentofacial Orthop*, 1987. **91**(3): p. 233–239.

43 Dewel, B.F., Clinical observations on the axial inclination of teeth. *Am J Orthod*, 1949. **35**(2): p. 98–115.

44 Tong, H., D. Kwon, J. Shi, N. Sakai, R. Enciso, and G.T. Sameshima, Mesiodistal angulation and faciolingual inclination of each whole tooth in 3-dimensional space in patients with near-normal occlusion. *Am J Orthod Dentofacial Orthop*, 2012. **141**(5): p. 604–617.

45 Al-Mashhadany, S.M., J.E. Saloom, and M. Nahidh, The relation among teeth and maxillary dental arch dimensions with anterior teeth angulation and inclination. *Sci World J*, 2021. **2021**: p. 8993734.

46 O'Higgins, E.A., R.H. Kirschen, and R.T. Lee, The influence of maxillary incisor inclination on arch length. *Br J Orthod*, 1999. **26**(2): p. 97–102.

47 Pontes, L.F., R.L. Cecim, S.M. Machado, and D. Normando, Tooth angulation and dental arch perimeter-the effect of orthodontic bracket prescription. *Eur J Orthod*, 2015. **37**(4): p. 435–439.

48 Verma, S., S. Singh, and A. Utreja, A normative study to evaluate inclination and angulation of teeth in North Indian population and comparison of expression of torque in preadjusted appliances. *J Orthod Sci*, 2014. **3**(3): p. 81–88.

3

Inter-arch Tooth Alignment

3.1   Introduction

The interrelation of the teeth in one arch to the teeth in the antagonistic arch is known as inter-arch tooth alignment. As the mandible closure happens, the maxillary and mandibular arches come into contact (Figure 3.1). The normal inter-arch relationship of the maxillary and mandibular teeth during occlusion is illustrated in this chapter.

3.2   Dental Occlusion

A condition where the teeth of both the mandible and maxilla are in contact is known to be occlusion. According to the Glossary of Prosthodontic Terms 9 (GPT-9), dental occlusion is (i) the process or the act of closure of the maxillary and mandibular arches, or (ii) the static relationship between the maxillary or mandibular teeth [1]. It indicates the static relationship between the arches. However, the teeth move in function over each other, and articulation/dynamic occlusion is established.

Different cusps, sulci, and grooves make the teeth' occlusal surfaces. The occlusal table is the region between the lingual and buccal cusp tip of the premolars and molars as shown in Figure 3.2 and it is approximately 50–60% of the buccolingual width [2].

It has been found that there exist differences in the occlusal form and cuspal tips in different populations [3]. According to a study of the Dutch population [3], the first upper molars cusps and ridges were higher in the Dutch population than those of the Japanese population, but distances between cuspal tips were smaller. According to another study [4], the molar cuspal heights were lower in Australian Aboriginals than in Dutch (Caucasoid) but higher than in Japanese (Mongoloid) populations. Intercuspal distances were considerably larger in Australian Aboriginals than those in the two other populations: Japanese (Mongoloid) and Dutch (Caucasoid). The differences in occlusal form can influence jaw movements in the two populations.

The region of a tooth that contacts the antagonistic teeth in the centric occlusion (CO) intercuspal position (ICP), and aids in the stability of occlusion, is termed the centric stop [2, 5]. For instance, the central fossa (central stop) of the mandibular first molar is contacted by the supporting cusp (mesiolingual cusp) of the maxillary first molar [5]. During the occlusal contacts,

Introduction to the Masticatory System and Dental Occlusion, First Edition. Dinesh Rokaya.
© 2025 John Wiley & Sons Ltd. Published 2025 by John Wiley & Sons Ltd.

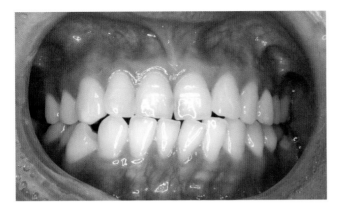

Figure 3.1 Teeth under occlusion in a natural dentition.

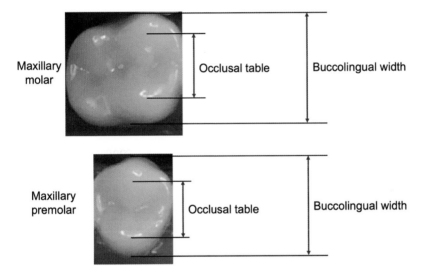

Figure 3.2 Occlusal table of the maxillary molar and premolar.

the occlusal forces must be aimed at the teeth's long axes and are important for obtaining occlusal stability in the ICP. The representation of ideal occlusal contacts is displayed in Figure 3.3. In order to maintain the occlusal stability that is needed for the success of orthodontic treatments, ideal occlusal contacts and localization of contacts in centric and eccentric occlusion should be considered [6]. Following orthodontic treatment, an increase in the number of occlusal contacts is usually desired during retention [7].

3.3 Overjet and Overbite

Typically, the mandibular arch is smaller than the maxillary arch. So, the maxillary teeth "overhang" the mandibular teeth during the CO/maximal intercuspation. The vertical overlap is called the overjet, and the horizontal (lateral or anteroposterior aspect) overlap

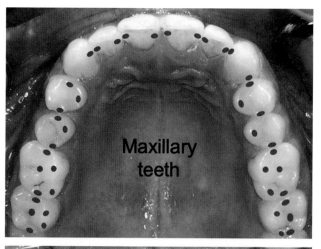

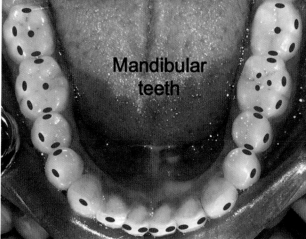

Figure 3.3 Ideal occlusal contacts, with marginal ridges and fossae of antagonistic teeth in the maxillary and mandibular arches.

is called the overbite (Figure 3.4) [2]. Normal overjet and overbite range from 2 to 4 mm [8]. Raj et al. [9] mentioned that the ideal overjet ranges from 1.5 to 2.5 mm and the ideal overbite range from 3 to 5 mm. There can be discrepancies in overjet and overbite during the mixed dentition period for temporary changes in the dentition [10]. These discrepancies will be compensated in part during mandibular growth and development of the dental arch.

The importance of overjet and overbite is related to mastication, speech, aesthetics, and jaw movements. Unnecessary vertical overlap of the anterior teeth can give rise to tissue impingement. It has been found that the overbite and overjet in an occlusion are not associated with any particular craniofacial pattern [11]. Fabian et al. [12] did a study to analyze the impact of overbite and overjet on the oral health-related quality of life of children and adolescents and they found that children and adolescents with overjet >6 mm are associated with significant limitations of the oral health-related quality of life. However, overbite deviations have only little impact on the oral health-related quality of life.

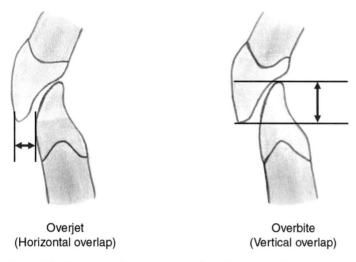

Overjet
(Horizontal overlap)

Overbite
(Vertical overlap)

Figure 3.4 Overjet (horizontal overlap of teeth) and overbite (vertical overlap of teeth).

3.4 Centric and Noncentric Cusps

The palatal cusps of maxillary posterior teeth and the buccal cusps of mandibular posterior teeth are called the centric/ functional/ supporting/ working cusps [2] as shown in Figures 3.5 and 3.6. These cusps occlude with the opposing central fossa and are crucial in keeping necessary space between the mandible and maxilla. These cusps have precise tips positioned nearly one-third the distance of the overall buccolingual width of the tooth.

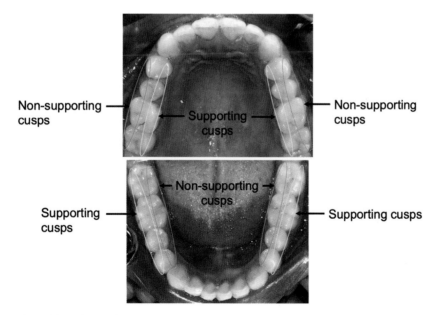

Figure 3.5 Supporting cusps (palatal cusps of maxillary posterior teeth and buccal cusps of mandibular posterior teeth) and nonsupporting cusps (buccal cusps of maxillary posterior teeth and lingual cusps of mandibular posterior teeth).

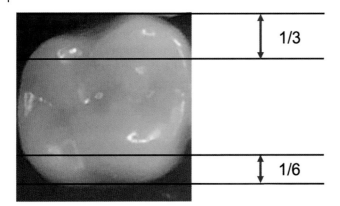

Figure 3.6 Supporting cusp (buccal cusps of mandibular posterior teeth showing one-third of the total buccolingual width) and nonsupporting cusp (lingual cusps of mandibular posterior teeth showing one-sixth of the total buccolingual width).

The buccal cusps of the maxillary posterior teeth and lingual cusps of mandibular posterior teeth are called noncentric/nonfunctional/nonsupporting/nonworking/guiding cusps [2]. These cusps have precise tips positioned nearly one-sixth the distance of the overall buccolingual width of the tooth. Since nonsupporting cusps contribute to food shearing during the process of mastication, they are also called shearing cusps. The noncentric cusps hold the food mass on the occlusal table for chewing and minimizing tissue impingement. They also maintain the stability of the mandible. A tight definite occlusal relationship is established when the teeth are in full occlusion.

Hwang et al. [13] studied the effects of orthodontic treatment on the centric discrepancy. They found that subjects with one prematurity were significantly greater in the control group (86.7%); nevertheless, subjects with >2 prematurities were greater in the orthodontic treatment group (41.6%) and showed more bilateral prematurities. There were no differences in centric prematurities. The centric prematurities were mostly seen on the buccal incline of the maxillary palatal cusp. This study showed that orthodontic treatment does not result in centric discrepancy normally. Similarly, He et al. [14] studied the relationship between centric relation-maximum intercuspation discrepancy and temporomandibular joint dysfunction (TMD) in pre-treated orthodontic patients and found that the centric relation-maximum intercuspation discrepancy can be a contributory factor to the development of TMD in patients.

3.5 Common Occlusal Relationships

3.5.1 Molar Classification

The molar relationship variations were first given by Angle [15] and consist of Angle class I–III molar relationship (Figures 3.7 and 3.8) [2].

Class I

Class II

Class III

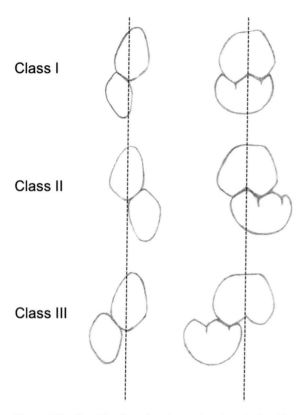

Figure 3.7 Classification of canine and molar relationships.

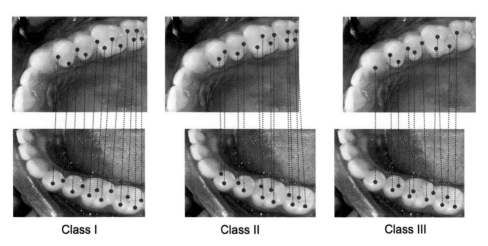

Class I   Class II   Class III

Figure 3.8 Contact areas occlusal seen in various molar relationships.

Class I: The class I molar relation is commonly seen in natural dentition. It is characterized as follows:
- Maxillary first molar's mesiobuccal cusp occludes on the buccal groove of the mandibular first molar.
- Maxillary first molar's mesiolingual cusp occludes in the central fossa region of the mandibular first molar.

Class II: In class II molar relation, the mandibular arch is found to be small in size or posteriorly placed, while the maxillary arch is found to be large or forwardly placed. It is characterized as follows:
- Maxillary first molar's distolingual cusp occludes in the C-F area of the mandibular first molar and mandibular first molar's mesiobuccal cusp occludes in the C-F area of the maxillary first molar.
- Mandibular first molar's mesiobuccal cusp occludes on the buccal groove of the maxillary first molar.

Class II division 1: Protrusion of maxillary incisors.
Class II division 2: Lingual inclination of maxillary incisors.
Class III: In molar class III molar relation, there is predominant growth of the mandible. It is characterized as follows:
- Maxillary first molar's mesiobuccal cusp is positioned over the embrasure between the mandibular first and second molar.
- Maxillary first molar's mesiolingual cusp is positioned in the mesial pit of the mandibular second molar.

A study by Alkayyal et al. [16] showed that patients with Angle's class I occlusion showed the most balanced occlusion, the least occlusion time, and a higher frequency of canine guidance. However, potentially balanced occlusion and group function were highly prevalent in all groups. Therefore, ideal occlusion is what is aimed for but cannot be considered a fundamental requirement of every dental treatment.

The class II and class III occlusion differ slightly from class I. In class II patients, the anterior teeth do not provide protection and guidance [17]. The posterior teeth bear the force from the occlusion. The most used and dominant movement is the protrusive movement. Most of the posterior teeth exhibit balancing contacts (bilateral balanced occlusion). The controlling factors are the posterior determinants of occlusion. Greater interocclusal clearance and adequate space during speech and function must be provided.

The class III jaw relations patient shows challenges in the occlusal patterns [18]. The lack of anterior guidance and increased length of the mandible have effects on occlusal morphology. Several stable forms of occlusal relationships can be found at one time in the same dentition. The occlusal morphology is guided by the condylar movements. The balancing cusps must provide proprioceptive guidance for the chewing cycle. About 1 mm of rest interocclusal distance is adequate to allow the teeth to separate during function and speech.

3.5.2 Canine Classification

Canine relationship, in a similar fashion to the molar relationship, is classified as class I, class II, and class III as shown in Figure 3.7.

Class I: In class I canine relation, the permanent maxillary canine directly occludes in the embrasure between the mandibular canine and first premolar.

Class II: In class II canine relation, the permanent maxillary canine occludes anterior to the embrasure between the mandibular canine and first premolar.

Class III: In class III canine relation, the permanent maxillary canine occludes posterior to the embrasure between the mandibular canine and first premolar.

3.5.3 Incisor Classification

The incisor relationship can be classified based on the Angle classification (Figure 3.9) [2]. This classification is based on the interrelation of the incisor tip of the mandible to the cingulum plateau of the central incisors of the maxilla.

Class I: In class I incisor relation, the incisor tips of the mandible occlude or rest beneath the cingulum plateau of the maxillary incisors.

Class II: In class II incisor relation, the incisor tips of the mandible occlude or rest posterior to the cingulum plateau of the maxillary incisors. It is additionally subdivided into:

Class II division 1: Increased overjet with straight or proclined maxillary incisors.

Class II division 2: Normal or increased overjet with retroclined maxillary incisors.

Class III: In class III incisor relation, the incisor tips of the mandible occlude or rest anterior to the cingulum plateau of the maxillary incisors.

Olliver et al. [19] did a longitudinal cohort study to investigate the changes in incisor relationships over three decades from adolescence to mid-adulthood, and they mentioned that the overjet values are found to be greater during mid-adulthood than during adolescence, while the converse is true for overbite. Incisor relationships change during the life course and are related to aging, periodontal health, gender, and parafunctional habits. The treatment decisions should follow the changes that occur in the incisor relationships.

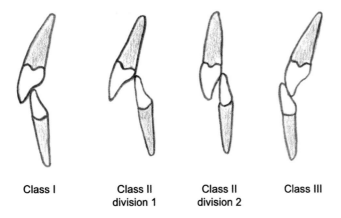

Class I Class II Class II Class III
     division 1 division 2

Figure 3.9 Classification of incisor relationship.

3.6 Position of Mandible and Condyle

The temporomandibular joint (TMJ) is a synovial hinge joint. It is at the junction of the mandibular head to the mandibular fossa and the temporal bone's articular tubercle (Figure 3.10) [2, 20]. Typically, two movements happen in the TMJ. First is the rotation movement where the mandibular head rotates anteriorly, and second is the translation movement where the mandibular head glides anteriorly while the rotation continues.

Various mandibular movements away from the CO ICP occur inside the envelope of border movements, such as protrusive, retrusive, lateral, and lateral protrusive. The lateral movements can be either on the left or the right.

3.6.1 Centric Relation

Centric relation can be described as maxillary and mandibular interrelation where the condyles articulate in the anterior-superior location against the articular eminence's posterior slopes. The CR is a reference position used clinically that is repeatable, and in this position, there only occurs rotational movement. The patients can make movements (lateral, vertical, or protrusive) from this unstrained, physiologic, and maxillomandibular relationship (GPT-9) [1].

3.6.2 Centric Occlusion

CO is the position of the jaw where the maxillary and mandibular teeth are in maximum contact or intercuspation (MI). CO is the occlusion most often used during mastication and it is also the occlusion for which the masticatory forces are the greatest [21]. Contacts in CO do not correspond to any ideal occlusion.

When the jaw is moved from the CR to initial contact (CR contact), typically one or two premature contacts occur. This usually occurs on the mesial cusp ridge of the upper first premolar or the oblique ridge of the upper molar. This movement from the premature contact in CR to the CO is known as the slide in centric. Both the ICP and CO are the

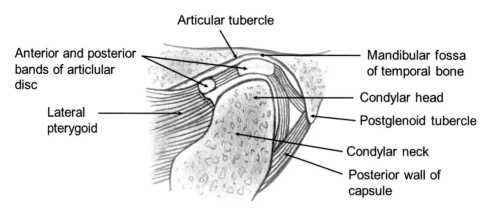

Figure 3.10 The anatomy of the condyle and temporomandibular joint. Adapted from Reference [20]; Copyright The Korean Society of Plastic and Reconstructive Surgeons (2012).

maximal intercuspation. The capability of closure into the MI in the absence of any interference between CO and CR is termed as freedom in centric. Selective grinding is the solution for the removal of any sort of interference in CR contact.

3.6.3   Vertical Dimension of Occlusion

The VDO is also called the occlusal vertical dimension (OVD), which is the distance between two specifically noted anatomical points during maximum intercuspation, i.e. the nose tip and the chin (Figure 3.11). In the case of teeth wear, a reduction in the OVD can be observed.

3.6.4   Vertical Dimension of Rest

The VDR is also known as the rest vertical dimension (RVD). It is the distance between two specific marked anatomical points at which a person is in an upright rest position. In this position, the muscles are in a minimal contracture position (Figure 3.11). This is known as the mandibular rest position and most of the mandibular movements start from this position.

3.6.5   Freeway Space

Freeway space is also called interocclusal space. It is the space between the maxillary and mandibular teeth when the mandible is in the rest position (Figure 3.11). Normally, it is around 2–3 mm.

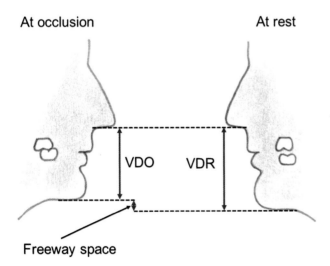

Figure 3.11   Vertical dimension at occlusion (VDO), vertical dimension at rest (VDR), and freeway space.

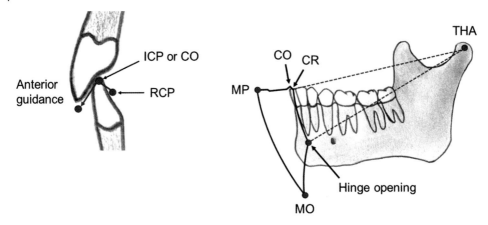

Figure 3.12 Envelope of mandibular movement in the sagittal plane. ICP = Intercuspal position, CO = Centric occlusion, RCP = Retruded contact position, CR = Centric relation, MP = Maximum protrusion, MO = Maximum opening, THA = Terminal hinge axis.

3.7 Terminal Hinge Axis Position and Retruded Contact Position

When there is retrusion of the mandible, the jaw interrelation of the mandible and maxilla in this position is denoted by CR. During the moment, when the mandible is backward and upward in a retrusive position, it is described as its most comfortable position. After this, the mandible gets opened and closed on an arc, and across the center of both the condylar heads an imaginary axis may be drawn described as the terminal hinge axis (THA) and it is the most reproducible jaw relationship (Figure 3.12) [2]. The first tooth contact when there is the closure of the mandible in the THA position is known as the retruded contact position (RCP). Approximately 1–2 mm of glide of the mandible and teeth from RCP to the ICP in an anterior and upward pathway is found in most patients.

3.8 Working and Nonworking (Balancing) Side

The mandible is lowered and there is a separation of the dental arches during the course of lateral movement (right side) (Figure 3.13) [2]. On the right working side, there is a movement of the jaw to the right, and at certain points right to the ICP/CO, the contact of teeth occurs. On the nonworking side (left side), there is either contact or no contact with the teeth. The movement of the condyle on the working side is called a laterotrusive movement (Figure 3.14) and that on the nonworking side is called mediotrusive movement [1, 2].

Not just the contact at the canine as in canine guidance but the multiple contact during lateral mandibular movements is called a group function. The contact of the anterior teeth in the course of protrusive mandibular movement is denoted as incisal guidance. It suggests that there are no differences in the dental occlusal that clearly separate asymptomatic from symptomatic patients with temporomandibular disorders [22]. The other guidance i.e. condylar and neuromuscular, are discussed later.

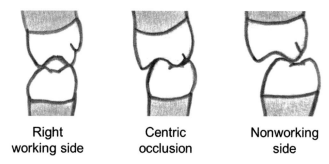

Right working side   Centric occlusion   Nonworking side

Figure 3.13 Contact relations of first molars (right side) of maxilla and mandible: right working side, centric occlusion, and nonworking side. Adapted from Reference [5]; chapter published in Wheeler's Dental Anatomy, Physiology, and Occlusion, 10th edition, Jelson S.J., Occlusion, page 285, Copyright Elsevier (2015).

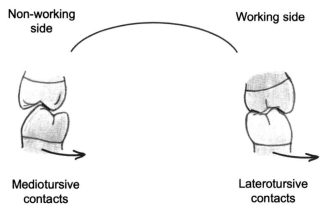

Non-working side   Working side

Mediotursive contacts   Laterotursive contacts

Figure 3.14 Left laterotrusive movement.

3.9 Tooth Guidance

Different forms of contact relations may be seen in the natural dentition, such as canine disocclusion, group function, or some blend of contacts in a molar, premolar, and canine during lateral mandibular movements.

3.9.1 Anterior or Lateral Guidance

The mandibular movements in the anterior region are controlled by the anterior teeth while that of the posterior region is controlled by the condyles. The lingual surfaces of the maxillary anterior teeth are contacted by the incisal edges of the lower teeth during the lateral or protrusive mandibular movement.

Anterior guidance is the influence of the contacting surfaces of anterior teeth, limiting mandibular movements (GPT 9) [1]. It is a highly variable factor. The contacting region of the maxillary and mandibular anterior teeth, the lingual surfaces' angle of the maxillary incisors, and the incisal path inclination (IPI) determine the mandibular movement in the

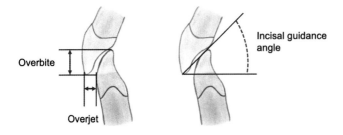

Figure 3.15 Overjet, overbite, and incisal guidance angle.

vertical direction. The incisal guidance has a horizontal component (overjet) and a vertical (overbite) component (Figure 3.15). The inclination level should be determined by the dentist, such as for aesthetic considerations. Likewise, the articulator motions are affected by the guidance table and pin.

The lingual surfaces of maxillary teeth are contacted by the incisal edges of the lower teeth in the course of lateral or protrusive movements. The vertical movement of the mandible is influenced by the inclination of the lingual surfaces. Dental procedures can help to change the anterior guidance. The two different parts can be used to evaluate the IPI.

3.9.1.1 Sagittal Protrusive Incisal Path Inclination

The IPI angle or the anterior guidance angle is formed in the sagittal plane between the occlusal line and the occlusal plane. During the moment when the teeth are in CO, the angle is formed between the horizontal plane and the line formed between the incisal edges of the mandibular and maxillary incisors in the sagittal plane (Figure 3.12). The IPI angle emerges via the vertical overlap (overbite) but depends on the amount of horizontal overlap (overjet) (Figure 3.16). A rise in the overjet results in a decrease of the IPI angle along with mandibular movement's vertical component and flattened posterior tubercles. Likewise, a rise in the overbite results in an increase in the IPI angle.

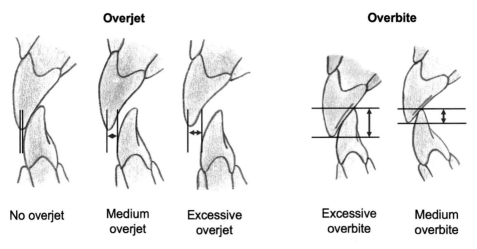

Figure 3.16 Different levels of overjet and overbite.

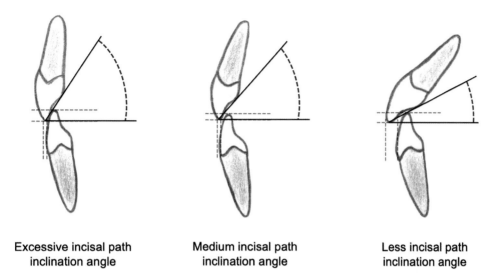

| Excessive incisal path inclination angle | Medium incisal path inclination angle | Less incisal path inclination angle |

Figure 3.17 Change of incisal path inclination angle with different levels of overjet and overbite.

So, the level of the vertical and horizontal overlaps decided by the teeth position in the case of dentures are completely managed by the dentists (Figure 3.16). In order to form the angle on the sagittal plane, the anterior guidance table in the articulator is referenced. Some of the various limitations of the IPI include arch shape, crest relations, crest width, and inter-crest distance. The patient's aesthetic and phonetic needs are tried to be fulfilled by the dentist creating the change in the IPI angle.

The level of horizontal and vertical overlaps is linked with the IPI (Figure 3.17). Decreasing the overbite will decrease the IPI angle. For example, if the amount of overbite is the same, the IPI might be adjusted by decreasing or increasing the horizontal overlap. The alignment of the mandibular incisors is near the lingual side, while the alignment of the maxillary incisors is near the vestibule (or both). The patient's aesthetic appearance should be considered in all of these processes.

In situations where a specific level of horizontal overlap is required, it's detrimental to raise the IPI via raising the vertical overlap as it can result in lateral forces that can injure the nearby tissues. Nevertheless, when the IPI reduces and slants near zero degrees, there is a rise in the stability of the denture. But the IPI along with the other factors should be adjusted while the denture stability and aesthetic appearance are properly considered.

3.9.1.2 Lateral Incisal Path Inclination
It is the angle formed between the horizontal plane and the path accompanied by the incisors and canines of the maxilla in the course of mandibular lateral movement that is known as lateral IPI. It involves the interrelation of incisors and canines.

3.9.2 Canine Guidance

Canine guidance, also known as canine-protected articulation, is a form of mutually protected occlusion in which the horizontal and vertical overlap of the canine discludes the posterior teeth in the excursive mandibular movements (GPT-9) [1].

Woda et al. [21] mentioned that canine protection and group function appear to correspond to two successive states of the evolving dentition under the effect of abrasion. In most lateral occlusions, two maxillary teeth, of which one is the canine, are involved.

3.10 Tooth Contacts

Teeth contact occurs during mastication and the contact occurs most often during a sliding movement in which the direction and the origin are variable [21]. During unilateral mastication, the chewing of the food is performed by working as well as nonworking contact. The occlusal contracts during swallowing are largely contradictory. The tooth can be examined clinically on patients, on casts, or on digital models (Figure 3.18) [23]. Digital casts can be used for quantification of the total occlusal contact area (in mm^2) owing to the high reliability of repeated measurements and the strong validity of the method compared to traditionally employed stone cast measurements.

3.10.1 Protrusive Contacts

During the protrusion, there is depression and anterior movement of the mandible that directs the anterior teeth together at positions that are suitable for incising food (Figure 3.19A) [2].

3.10.2 Retrusive Contacts

Retrusive movement happens when there is a posterior movement of the mandible through the ICP [2]. This movement is a bit small (1–2 mm) as it is confined by the ligamentous structures (Figure 3.19B).

Riise and Ericsson [24] did a clinical study of the distribution of occlusal tooth contacts in molars, premolars, and anterior teeth in the ICP during light and hard pressure in young adults (Md 24) and adults (Md 41). They found that there was no difference between the right and left side and the number of contacts per tooth. In all teeth, there was a smaller number of contacts at light pressure. The lower number of contacts at light pressure (in anterior teeth) is seen in adults when compared with young adults. There was an increase in the number of contacts at hard pressure which was greater for the anterior teeth than for the molars.

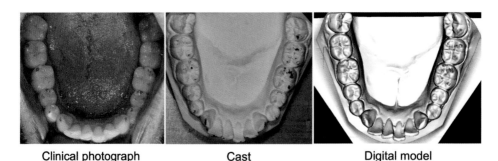

Clinical photograph   Cast   Digital model

Figure 3.18 Examination of occlusal contacts clinically, on cast, and digitally. Reproduced from Reference [23] / with permission of John Wiley & Sons.

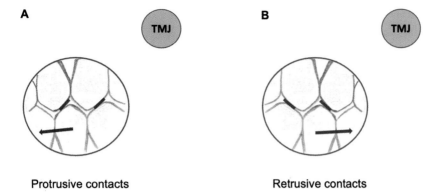

Protrusive contacts   Retrusive contacts

Figure 3.19 Posterior protrusive and retrusive contacts. A, Posterior protrusive contacts (distal inclines of the maxillary teeth and the mesial inclines of the mandibular teeth). B, Posterior retrusive contacts (mesial inclines of the maxillary teeth and the distal inclines of the mandibular teeth).

Finally, there is no standardization of occlusal contact type and various factors influence the number of occlusal contacts between a class I and class II occlusal relationship [25]. A proper selection of occlusal contact types should be done, i.e. cusps to fossa or cusps to the marginal ridge, and their location in the teeth should be individually defined according to the need of each case. Good occlusal contact results in the correct distribution of forces and good periodontal health.

3.11 Occlusal Contact and Stability

Occlusal stability indicates the status of the muscles, jaws, teeth, and joints to stay in an optimally functional state [5]. The pressure from the lip, cheek, and tongue, the occlusal forces, and the support from the periodontium are engaged in maintaining the stability of the teeth position and the occlusion. If there are changes in frequency, magnitude, or duration, the stability is disturbed and the teeth may drift, disrupting the occlusion. Loss of tooth, tooth structure, supporting cusps, the reduction in periodontal support, and trauma can affect occlusal stability. These may result in the migration of teeth mesially, supra eruption of teeth, wear via occlusal forces, bone remodeling, control of occlusal forces, and reparative processes. Hence, to maintain occlusal stability, occlusal therapy should be done which includes preservation of a stable CR and CO, occlusal force direction on the long axis of the tooth, preservation of supporting cusps, centric stops, VD, replacement of missing teeth, and management of mobile teeth.

Mesial migration is the movement of teeth toward the mesial direction. The reasons involve transseptal fiber traction, masticatory forces, and tongue pressure [26–29]. The proximal tooth contacts' closure via occlusal forces may be related to the mesial migration.

Following the orthodontic treatment, increased occlusal contacts are usually desired during retention. Sauget et al. [7] compared the occlusal contacts in Hawley and clear overlay orthodontic retainers relative to changes in the number of occlusal contacts. The Hawley retainer showed a significant increase in occlusal contacts on posterior teeth and no change on anterior teeth. The Hawley retainer allows relative vertical movement of the posterior teeth which was not seen in the clear overlay retainer.

Finally, Estelle et al. [30] proposed a precise classification of occlusal functions to establish a positive diagnosis of occlusal disorders and presented three kinds of occlusal functions: stabilizing dysfunction, centering dysfunction, and guiding dysfunction. This occlusal function or dysfunction classification allows lines to be drawn between different occlusal situations, such as a loss of posterior occlusal support and loss of OVD, short or reduced dental arch, reversed and scissor occlusion, posterior occlusal interference and balancing contact, infra-occlusion, and loss of posterior support, sagittally, and transversely deflected mandible.

References

1 Ferro, K.J. The glossary of prosthodontic terms: ninth edition. *J Prosthet Dent*, 2017. **117**: p. e1–e105.

2 Okeson, J.P., *Management of Temporomandibular Disorders and Occlusion*. 7th ed. 2013, St. Louis, Missouri: Mosby.

3 Kanazawa, E., M. Sekikawa, and T. Ozaki, Three-dimensional measurements of the occlusal surfaces of upper molars in a Dutch population. *J Dent Res*, 1984. **63**(11): p. 1298–1301.

4 Sekikawa, M., J. Akai, E. Kanazawa, and T. Ozaki, Three-dimensional measurement of the occlusal surfaces of lower first molars of Australian aboriginals. *Am J Phys Anthropol*, 1986. **71**(1): p. 25–32.

5 Nelson, S.J., *Wheeler's Dental Anatomy, Physiology, and Occlusion*. 10th ed. 2015, St. Louis, Missouri: Saunders.

6 Dinçer, M., O. Meral, and N. Tümer, The investigation of occlusal contacts during the retention period. *Angle Orthod*, 2003. **73**(6): p. 640–646.

7 Sauget, E., D.A. Covell, Jr., R.P. Boero, and W.S. Lieber, Comparison of occlusal contacts with use of Hawley and clear overlay retainers. *Angle Orthod*, 1997. **67**(3): p. 223–230.

8 Kinaan, B.K., Overjet and overbite distribution and correlation: a comparative epidemiological English-Iraqi study. *Br J Orthod*, 1986. **13**(2): p. 79–86.

9 Raj, A., R. Ranjan, A. Kumar, M. Kumar, N. Mala, and K. Ramesh, Evaluation of dental status in relation to excessive horizontal and vertical overlap in North Indian population. *J Pharm Bioallied Sci*, 2021. **13**(Suppl 1): p. S276–S279.

10 Tausche, E., O. Luck, and W. Harzer, Prevalence of malocclusions in the early mixed dentition and orthodontic treatment need. *Eur J Orthod*, 2004. **26**(3): p. 237–244.

11 Ioannidou, I., E. Gianniou, T. Koutsikou, and G. Kolokithas, Quantitative description of overjet and overbite and their relationship with the craniofacial morphology. *Clin Orthod Res*, 1999. **2**(3): p. 154–161.

12 Fabian, S., B. Gelbrich, A. Hiemisch, W. Kiess, and C. Hirsch, Impact of overbite and overjet on oral health-related quality of life of children and adolescents. *J Orofac Orthop*, 2018. **79**(1): p. 29–38.

13 Hwang, H.S. and R.G. Behrents, The effect of orthodontic treatment on centric discrepancy. *Cranio*, 1996. **14**(2): p. 132–137.

14 He, S.S., X. Deng, P. Wamalwa, and S. Chen, Correlation between centric relation–maximum intercuspation discrepancy and temporomandibular joint dysfunction. *Acta Odontol Scand*, 2010. **68**(6): p. 368–376.

15 Angle, E.H., Classification of malocclusion. *Dent Cosmos*, 1899. **41**: p. 248–264.

16 Alkayyal, M.A., K.A. Turkistani, A.A. Al-Dharrab, M.A. Abbassy, M. Melis, and K.H. Zawawi, Occlusion time, occlusal balance and lateral occlusal scheme in subjects with various dental and skeletal characteristics: a prospective clinical study. *J Oral Rehabil*, 2020. **47**(12): p. 1503–1510.

17 Jensen, W.O., Occlusion for the Class II jaw relations patient. *J Prosthet Dent*, 1990. **64**(4): p. 432–434.

18 Jensen, W.O., Occlusion for the Class III jaw relations patient. *J Prosthet Dent*, 1990. **64**(5): p. 566–568.

19 Olliver, S.J., J.M. Broadbent, S. Prasad, C. Cai, W.M. Thomson, and M. Farella, Changes in incisor relationship over the life course - findings from a cohort study. *J Dent*, 2022. **117**: p. 103919.

20 Choi, K.-Y., J.D. Yang, H.-Y. Chung, and B.-C. Cho, Current concepts in the mandibular condyle fracture management part I: overview of condylar fracture. *Arch Plast Surg*, 2012. **39**: p. 291–300.

21 Woda, A., P. Vigneron, and D. Kay, Nonfunctional and functional occlusal contacts: a review of the literature. *J Prosthet Dent*, 1979. **42**(3): p. 335–341.

22 Kahn, J., R.H. Tallents, R.W. Katzberg, M.E. Ross, and W.C. Murphy, Prevalence of dental occlusal variables and intraarticular temporomandibular disorders: molar relationship, lateral guidance, and nonworking side contacts. *J Prosthet Dent*, 1999. **82**(4): p. 410–415.

23 Sigvardsson, J., S. Nilsson, M. Ransjö, and A. Westerlund, Digital quantification of occlusal contacts: a methodological study. *Int J Environ Res Public Health*, 2021. **18**(10): p. 5297.

24 Riise, C. and S.G. Ericsson, A clinical study of the distribution of occlusal tooth contacts in the intercuspal position at light and hard pressure in adults. *J Oral Rehabil*, 1983. **10**(6): p. 473–480.

25 Watanabe-Kanno, G.A. and J. Abrão, Study of the number of occlusal contacts in maximum intercuspation before orthodontic treatment subjects with Angle Class I and Class II Division 1 malocclusion. *Dental Press J Orthod*, 2012. **17**(1): p. 138–147.

26 Picton, D.C. and J.P. Moss, The effect on approximal drift of altering the horizontal component of biting force in adult monkeys (macaca irus). *Arch Oral Biol*, 1980. **25**(1): p. 45–48.

27 van Beek, H. and V.J. Fidler, An experimental study of the effect of functional occlusion on mesial tooth migration in macaque monkeys. *Arch Oral Biol*, 1977. **22**(4): p. 269–271.

28 Dewel, B.F., Clinical observations on the axial inclination of teeth. *Am J Orthod*, 1949. **35**(2): p. 98–115.

29 Yilmaz, R.S., A.I. Darling, and B.G. Levers, Mesial drift of human teeth assessed from ankylosed deciduous molars. *Arch Oral Biol*, 1980. **25**(2): p. 127–231.

30 Estelle, C., R. Jean-Philippe, G. Anne, P. Anne, and O. Jean-Daniel, Dental occlusion: proposal for a classification to guide occlusal analysis and optimize research protocols. *J Contemp Dent Pract*, 2021. **22**(7): p. 840–849.

4

Occlusal Surface of Teeth and Characteristics of Jaw Movement

4.1 Introduction

The occlusal anatomy of teeth and the structures controlling the mandible's pattern of movement should be in balance with each other. Two structures control the mandibular movement: (i) those that influence the movement of the posterior portion of the mandible, and (ii) those that influence the movement of the anterior portion of the mandible [1]. The temporomandibular joints (TMJs) are the posterior controlling factors and the anterior teeth are the anterior controlling factors [2]. The posterior teeth are positioned between these two controlling factors and are affected by both to varying degrees [2, 3]. In patients, it is important to examine these structures that make up the occlusal plane, as well as their positioning in order to achieve an optimal occlusal relationship and to achieve the best functional relationship with the TMJs [1].

From the point of view of occlusion, the appearance of the incisors marks for the first time the conformation of an occlusal tripodism, given by the anterior teeth and the TMJs [1]. From this moment on, important anatomical and functional changes begin to take place, basically the development of the zygomatic tubercle before the modification of mandibular movements, which have become more complex cycles that include vertical, lateral, and protrusive movements.

4.2 Posterior Controlling Factors (Condylar Guidance)

When there is a condylar movement through the centric relation position, it moves across the mandibular fossa's articular eminence and this motion is dependent on the articular eminence inclination [2]. If there is a sharp inclination of the articular eminence, the condyle follows a vertically inclined path, and if there is a flat articular eminence, the condyle follows a less vertically inclined path. Furthermore, the condylar guidance angle is formed between the movement of the condyle apart and the horizontal reference plane [2, 4, 5]. Condylar guidance is usually fixed as it cannot be altered in healthy patients; however, it can be altered in specific cases (trauma or pathosis).

Dewan et al. [4] compared the condylar guidance by the conventional method using interocclusal records and panoramic radiographs and they found that there was a significant difference between the two methods. The condylar guidance values obtained from the interocclusal record method were less when compared to the values obtained from the radiographic method (tracing the panoramic radiographs). The radiograph method using panoramic X-ray to measure the condylar guidance can be an alternative to an interocclusal recording method for determining the condylar guidance in dentate and edentulous conditions [6].

Motoyoshi et al. [7] studied the condylar path angle in relation to Angle's classification with the overbite and subjective symptoms and found that the condylar path angle in Angle's class I group was similar to that in Angle's class II, whereas in Angle's class III, the condylar path angle was smaller than in class I and class II. Furthermore, they also found that the condylar path angle was decreased in a smaller overbite. In the symptom group, the condylar path angle was slightly smaller than in the nonsymptom group. This observation can be explained by a disorder of the control mechanism of the anterior and posterior factors. When the posterior control factor is steep, the condyle does not show harmony with its motion, and it can result in a molar disclusion [7]. In addition, when the condylar path angle is too small, it often results in occlusal interference in the posterior teeth.

4.3 Anterior Controlling Factors (Anterior Guidance)

Anterior movement of the mandible is determined by the anterior teeth. The lingual surfaces of the maxillary teeth come in contact with the mandibular teeth' incisal edges when there is a protrusion or lateral mandibular movement [2]. Vertical mandibular movement is ascertained by the inclination of the maxillary anterior teeth's lingual surfaces. Steep surfaces describe the mandibular anterior portion as having a steeply inclined path, however, if there is a slight vertical overlap (VO) of the anterior teeth, then they might have less vertical guidance [2, 8].

The anterior teeth protect the posterior teeth by resulting in disocclusion of the posterior in eccentric positions. Similarly, the posterior teeth protect the anterior teeth by taking most forces during closure in a centric position. The anterior guidance is a result of both anterior tooth position and condylar border movements; both factors must be considered in the creation of an anterior guidance [8]. The anterior guidance is important in oral rehabilitation [9, 10] and it is not fixed, so, it may be altered via dental treatments (orthodontics, restorations, and extractions) and pathological conditions (tooth wear, habits, and caries).

The occlusal surfaces of the posterior teeth have cusps formed of convex ridges which differ in vertical inclination and horizontal direction. There is a close relationship between these components and the mandibular movement in a superoinferior and anteroposterior direction. Furthermore, deficiencies in anterior guidance also give rise to posterior interference [7]. Both control factors function together to define jaw movement. Recently, the anterior guidance has been found to influence the working condylar path and can change the lateral incisal path [11]. This shows that the anterior guidance and condylar path are related and dependent factors.

4.4   Vertical Determinants of Occlusal Morphology

The vertical determinants of occlusal morphology have an impact on the cuspal height and fossae depths. The following three factors influence the length of the cusp and the distance of its extension in the fossa depth [2]:

1) Mandibular movement's anterior controlling factor (anterior guidance).
2) Mandibular movement's posterior controlling factor (condylar guidance).
3) Cusp nearness to those controlling factors.

During intercuspal position (ICP), the posterior centric contact, disoccludes in eccentric movements of the mandible. For this, posterior centric contact should be adequately long to make contact during the ICP; however, they should not be too long to do so in eccentric movements.

4.4.1   Effect of Condylar Guidance on Cusp Height

As mentioned before, when there is a protrusion of the mandible, the descent of the condyle through the articular eminence in regard to the horizontal plane is decided via the eminence's inclination [2, 12]. The steeper eminence causes larger vertical movement of the mandibular teeth, condyle, and mandible.

In Figure 4.1, there is a movement of the condyle at a 45° angle, away from the horizontal reference plane [2]. Premolar A's cusp tip shall shift away via a horizontal plane at a 45° angle. To avoid eccentric contact between the premolars in the protrusive movement, the cuspal inclination should be <45°.

4.4.2   Effect of Anterior Guidance on Cusp Height

The functional interrelation between the anterior teeth of the mandible and maxilla is known as anterior guidance [2]. It consists of the VO and horizontal overlap (HO) of the anterior teeth which influence the mandibular movements as shown in Figure 4.2 [2]. Since the anterior guidance greatly determines the mandibular movement, variation in the mandibular vertical movement pattern results from variation in VO and HO of the anterior teeth [12]. A rise in HO results in a reduction of mandibular movement's vertical component, flat posterior cusps, and a reduction of anterior guidance angle. A rise in VO results in an increase in mandibular movement's vertical component, steep posterior cusps, and greater anterior guidance angle.

4.4.3   Effect of Occlusion Pane on Cusp Height

An imaginary line that touches the anterior teeth's incisal edges and posterior teeth's cusps of the maxilla, respectively, is known as the occlusion plane (OP). The inclination of the cusps is determined by the interrelation of the OP to the angle of eminence. The OP's influence can be viewed during mandibular tooth movement that is seen in regards to the OP [2].

The anterior guidance, as well as condylar guidance, are united to bring out a 45° movement of the tooth of the mandible compared with the horizontal reference plane (Figure 4.3) [2]. Nevertheless, while comparing 45° movement with one OP$_A$, there is only

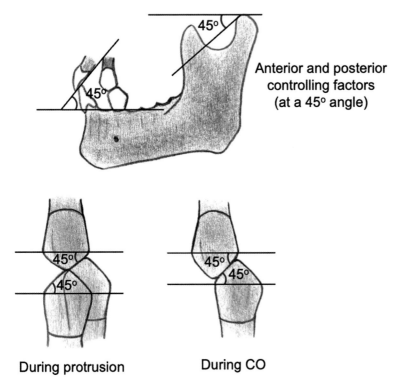

Anterior and posterior
controlling factors
(at a 45° angle)

During protrusion   During CO

Figure 4.1 Anterior controlling and posterior controlling factors resulting in the mandibular movement off the reference plane at a 45° angle. During protrusion, to disocclude one premolar from the other premolar, the cuspal inclines must be <45° angle. Adapted from Reference [2]; chapter published in Management of Temporomandibular Disorders and Occlusion, 7th edition, Okeson J.P., Determinants of Occlusion Morphology, page 89, Copyright Elsevier (2013).

a 25° angle movement of the tooth off the plane that causes a necessity of posterior cusps that are flatter, such that the contact of the posterior tooth might be averted. Also, while comparing the movement of the tooth with the next OP_B, it is 60° off this plane. Hence, the cusps of posterior teeth might be longer, and it is known that when OP turns out to be almost parallel to the angle of eminence, the posterior cusps need to be made shorter.

Furthermore, the anatomy of the cusps of posterior teeth should be in the appropriate form aligned to the condylar path so that it also contributes to the posterior disclusion [11]. Posterior disclusion is an important factor in controlling harmful lateral forces. The molars must disclude slightly more than the deviation in the condylar path in order to avoid occlusal interferences. The angle of hinge rotation created by the angular difference between anterior guidance and condylar path helps the posterior disclusion.

4.4.4 Effect of Curve of Spee on Cusp Height

The anteroposterior curve that extends from the mandibular canine tip along the mandibular posterior teeth's buccal cusp tips is known as the curve of Spee. The curve's radial length can be used to describe its curvature [13]. The curve is more acute with a short radius

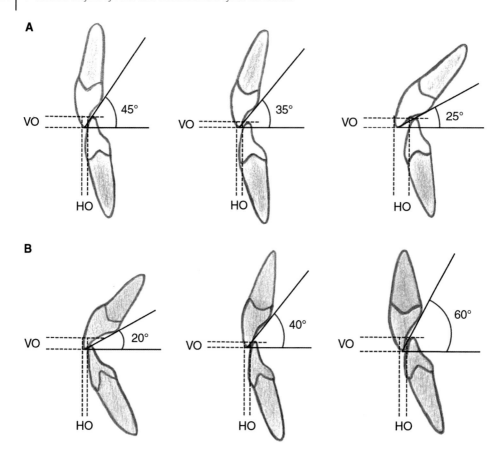

Figure 4.2 The alteration of anterior guidance angle through the variations in the vertical overlap (VO) and horizontal overlap (HO). A, An increase in HO decreases the anterior guidance angle at constant VO. B, An increase in VO increases the anterior guidance angle at constant HO. Adapted from Reference [2]; chapter published in Management of Temporomandibular Disorders and Occlusion, 7th edition, Okeson J.P., Determinants of Occlusion Morphology, page 90, Copyright Elsevier (2013).

rather than a long radius (Figure 4.4) [2]. A shorter radius for the arc of rotation of the mandibular dental arch results in deeper curved surfaces of the maxillary and mandibular dental arches [14]. In contrast, a larger radius for the arc of rotation of the mandibular dental arch results in shallower curved surfaces of the maxillary and mandibular dental arches.

The posterior cusp's height is influenced by the curve of Spee's curvature which shall function in balance with the mandibular movement. As the mandible moves off the horizontal reference plane at a 45° angle (Figure 4.5) [2], the posterior teeth's movement of the maxilla also varies relying on the curvature of the curve of Spee. Rather than with a longer radius, a greater angle is present with a shorter radius where the teeth of the mandible move away from the teeth of the maxilla. The curvature and orientation of the curve of Spee also influence the cusp height of posterior teeth (Figure 4.5) [2].

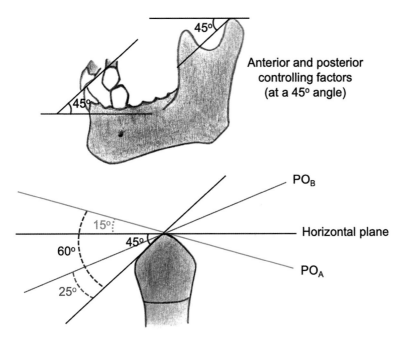

Anterior and posterior
controlling factors
(at a 45° angle)

PO_B

Horizontal plane

PO_A

Figure 4.3 Anterior controlling and posterior controlling factors. The mandibular movement of 45° via the horizontal plane is created through the anterior and posterior controlling factors. There is a movement of the tooth at a 45° angle through the reference plane. Nonetheless, if one occlusion plane (OP$_A$ is angled, there is a movement of the tooth of the reference plane at just 25°, so to disocclude during protrusive movement, the cusp should be reasonably flat. During the protrusive movement, the angle at which there is tooth movement, when compared with another occlusion plane (OP$_B$, a relatively greater discrepancy is visible (45 + 15 = 60°) that permits for more tall and steep posterior cusps. Adapted from Reference [2]; chapter published in Management of Temporomandibular Disorders and Occlusion, 7th edition, Okeson J.P., Determinants of Occlusion Morphology, page 91, Copyright Elsevier (2013).

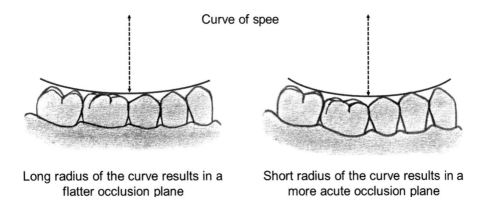

Curve of spee

Long radius of the curve results in a
flatter occlusion plane

Short radius of the curve results in a
more acute occlusion plane

Figure 4.4 Curve of Spee. The long radius of the curve results in a flatter occlusion plane, whereas the short radius of the curve results in a more acute occlusion plane. Adapted from Reference [2]; chapter published in Management of Temporomandibular Disorders and Occlusion, 7th edition, Okeson J.P., Determinants of Occlusion Morphology, page 91, Copyright Elsevier (2013).

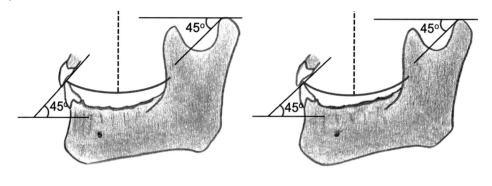

Flatter the plane of occlusion with taller teeth

More acute the plane of occlusion with shorter teeth

Figure 4.5 Occlusion plane and design. An acute occlusion plane results in a smaller angle of the movement of the mandible's posterior teeth, hence the cusps/teeth can be shorter. Hence, in the flatter plane of occlusion, the cusps/teeth can be taller. Adapted from Reference [2]; chapter published in Management of Temporomandibular Disorders and Occlusion, 7th edition, Okeson J.P., Determinants of Occlusion Morphology, page 92, Copyright Elsevier (2013).

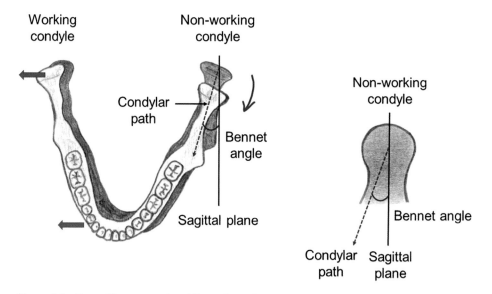

Figure 4.6 Bennett's movement and Bennet's angle.

4.4.5 Effect of Mandibular Lateral Translation Movement on Cusp Height

While the lateral movements of the mandible occur, the bodily shift of the mandible is called the mandibular lateral translation (Bennett movements) [15]. The angle created between the sagittal plane and the average path of the nonworking-side condyle in the horizontal plane, during lateral movements of the mandible, is known as Bennett's angle (Figure 4.6) [16]. Generally, Bennet's angle is about 7.5°–12.8°.

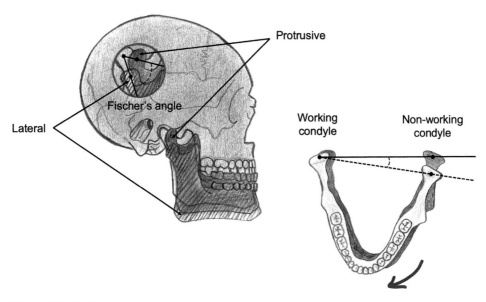

Figure 4.7 Fischer's angle.

Bennet angle $(L) = H/8 + 12$ (H = Horizontal condylar inclination).

The angle created by the inclination of working (orbiting) and nonworking side (rotating) condylar paths, as viewed from the sagittal plane, is called Fisher's angle (Figure 4.7) [17].

The orbiting condyle in the mandibular fossa in the course of a lateral excursion passes forward, downward, and inward around the axes situated in the opposite (rotating) condyle (Figure 4.8) [2]. There are two factors that determine the orbiting condyle's degree of inward movement: the mandibular fossa's medial wall's morphology and the temporomandibular ligament's (TML) inner horizontal part that attaches to the rotating condyle's lateral pole [2]. Mostly, some amount of relaxation of TML is present and the mandibular fossa's medial wall stays medial to an arc about the rotating condyle's axis.

There are three aspects of lateral translation movement: direction, amount, and timing. The degree to which the mandibular fossa's medial wall shifts medially about the axis in the rotating condyle by the ligament defines the amount and timing.

4.4.5.1 Effect of the Amount of Lateral Translation Movement on Cusp Height

The looser TML results in a greater quantity of translation movement of the mandible [2]. The mandible's bodily shift occurs when there is a rise in the lateral movement that is determined by the posterior cusps (Figure 4.9) [2].

4.4.5.2 Effect of the Direction of the Lateral Translation Movement on Cusp Height

The ligamentous attachments and morphology of the TMJ going through rotation determine the rotating condyle's direction of shift during a lateral translation [2]. The translation movement happens inside a <60° cone which has an apex positioned at the axis of rotation (Figure 4.10) [2]. So, besides the lateral movement, the rotating condyle can further move (i) anterior, (ii) posterior, (iii) superior, (iv) inferior direction, or a mixture of these.

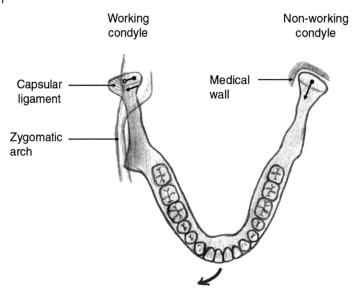

Figure 4.8 Mandibular lateral translation occurs due to the space between the orbiting condyle's medial pole and the medial wall, and some rotating condyle movement is permitted by the TML. Adapted from Reference [2]; chapter published in Management of Temporomandibular Disorders and Occlusion, 7th edition, Okeson J.P., Determinants of Occlusion Morphology, page 93, Copyright Elsevier (2013).

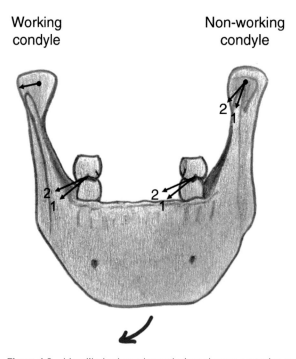

Figure 4.9 Mandibular lateral translation; shorter posterior cusp results in greater lateral translation movement. Progressive side shift (1). Immediate side shift (2). Adapted from Reference [2]; chapter published in Management of Temporomandibular Disorders and Occlusion, 7th edition, Okeson J.P., Determinants of Occlusion Morphology, page 94, Copyright Elsevier (2013).

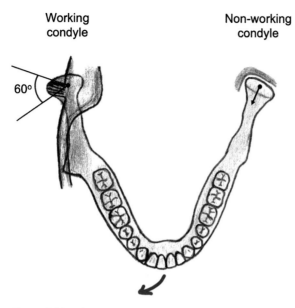

Working
condyle

Non-working
condyle

60°

Figure 4.10 The movement of the rotating condyle laterally inside the region of a 60° cone in the course of lateral translation movement. Adapted from Reference [2]; chapter published in Management of Temporomandibular Disorders and Occlusion, 7th edition, Okeson J.P., Determinants of Occlusion Morphology, page 94, Copyright Elsevier (2013).

In the course of a lateral translation, the rotating condyle's vertical movement is determined by the depth of the fossa and the height of the cusp (for example, the inferior and superior movements) (Figure 4.11) [2]. If the posterior cusps are shorter, it will result in a straight lateral movement in the rotating condyle's laterosuperior movement. And if the posterior cusps are longer, it will result in a straight lateral movement in lateroinferior movement.

4.4.5.3 Effect of the Timing of the Lateral Translation Movement on Cusp Height

The attachment of the TML to the rotating condyle and the medial wall near the orbiting condyle determines the lateral movement's timing [2]. In the early phase of laterotrusive movement, the occlusal morphology is remarkably influenced by the direction and amount of the lateral translation movement. A shift is noticed when there is an occurrence of early lateral translation movement, even prior to the start of translation of the condyle through the fossa, which is known as an immediate side shift or immediate lateral translation movement (Figure 4.12) [2]. When this happens in combination with an eccentric movement, then it is inferred as a progressive side shift or lateral translation movement. The shorter posterior cusp results in more immediate lateral translation.

4.5   Horizontal Determinants of Occlusal Morphology

The connections that influence the path of grooves and ridges on the occlusal surfaces are included in the horizontal determinants of occlusal morphology. The placement of cusps is also influenced by the horizontal determinants since the cusps course over grooves and

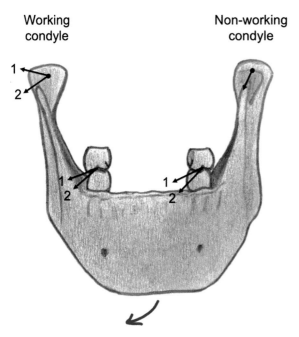

Figure 4.11 A Shorter posterior cusp results in a more superior rotating condyle's lateral translation movement (1). A taller posterior cusp results in more inferior lateral translation movement (2). Adapted from Reference [2]; chapter published in Management of Temporomandibular Disorders and Occlusion, 7th edition, Okeson J.P., Determinants of Occlusion Morphology, page 95, Copyright Elsevier (2013).

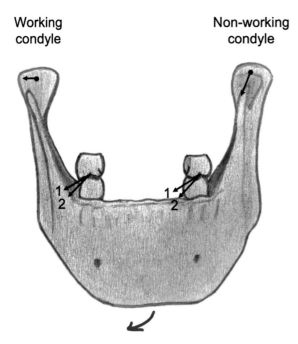

Figure 4.12 Lateral translation movement's timing. Immediate lateral movement (immediate side shift) (1). Progressive lateral movement (progressive side shift) (2). Adapted from Reference [2]; chapter published in Management of Temporomandibular Disorders and Occlusion, 7th edition, Okeson J.P., Determinants of Occlusion Morphology, page 95, Copyright Elsevier (2013).

between the ridges during eccentric movements. Both the mediotrusive and laterotrusive pathways are generated by each cusp tip through its opposite tooth and exhibit an arc portion made by the cusp that rotates around the rotating condyle. There is a variation of the angles made by these pathways relying on the correlation of the angle to specific anatomic structures.

4.5.1 Effect of Distance from the Condyle on Ridge and Groove Direction

When the tooth position differs in relation to the condyle's axis of rotation, the alteration can happen in the angles created by the pathways [2]. The farther the tooth from the axis of rotation (rotating condyle), the broader the angle created by the mediotrusive and laterotrusive pathways (Figure 4.13) [2]. Since the pathways of the mandible are being more mesially generated, there is an increase in the size of the angles when there is an increase in distance from the rotating condyle.

4.5.2 Effect of Distance from the Midsagittal Plane on Ridge and Groove Direction

The pathways on the tooth by an opposite centric cusp are also influenced by the interrelation of a tooth to the midsagittal plane. The angles made by the mediotrusive and laterotrusive pathways rise when the tooth is far from the midsagittal plane (Figure 4.14) [2].

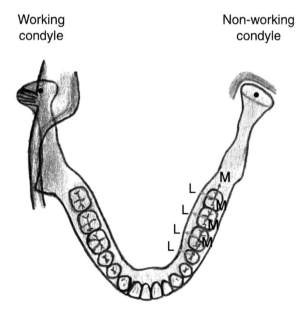

Figure 4.13 Greater the interspace between the tooth and the rotating condyle, the wider the angle made by the laterotrusive (L) and mediotrusive pathways (M). Adapted from Reference [2]; chapter published in Management of Temporomandibular Disorders and Occlusion, 7th edition, Okeson J.P., Determinants of Occlusion Morphology, page 96, Copyright Elsevier (2013).

Working
condyle

Non-working
condyle

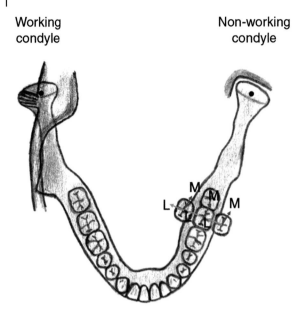

Figure 4.14 Greater the interspace between the tooth and the midsagittal plane, the wider the angle made by the laterotrusive (L) and mediotrusive (M) pathways. Adapted from Reference [2]; chapter published in Management of Temporomandibular Disorders and Occlusion, 7th edition, Okeson J.P., Determinants of Occlusion Morphology, page 96, Copyright Elsevier (2013).

4.6 Relationship Between Anterior and Posterior Controlling Factors

There is an interrelation between the condylar guidance's horizontal and vertical factors with that of maxillary anterior teeth' lingual concavities (anterior guidance's horizontal and vertical correlation) [2, 9]. The anterior guidance must be in harmony with the condylar guidance. When the movement of the condyle further goes horizontal, the articular eminence's angle decreases with a rise in lateral translation.

References

1 Puebla, R.L. and C.T.A. Soto, The role of the occlusal plane in joint health in orthodontic diagnosis (Part I). *Rev Mex Ortodon*, 2020. **8**(1): p. 60–68.

2 Okeson, J.P., *Management of Temporomandibular Disorders and Occlusion*. 7th ed. 2013, St. Louis, Missouri: Mosby.

3 Ricketts, R.M., Variations of the temporomandibular joint as revealed by cephalometric laminagraphy. *Am J Orthod*, 1950. **36**(12): p. 877–898.

4 Dewan, H., T.I. Akkam, H. Chohan, A. Sherwani, F. Masha, and M. Dhae, Comparison of sagittal condylar guidance determined by panoramic radiographs to the one determined by conventional methods using lateral interocclusal records in the Saudi Arabian population. *J Int Soc Prev Community Dent*, 2019. **9**(6): p. 597–604.

 5 Aull, A.E., Condylar determinants of occlusal patterns. *J Prosthet Dent*, 1965. **15**(5): p. 826–849.

 6 Godavarthi, A.S., M.C. Sajjan, A.V. Raju, P. Rajeshkumar, A. Premalatha, and N. Chava, Correlation of condylar guidance determined by panoramic radiographs to one determined by conventional methods. *J Int Oral Health*, 2015. **7**(8): p. 123–128.

 7 Motoyoshi, M., K. Inoue, K. Kiuchi, M. Ohya, A. Nakajima, T. Aramoto, and S. Namura, Relationships of condylar malocclusion and temporomandibular joint disturbances. *J Nihon Univ Sch Dent*, 1993. **35**: p. 43–48.

 8 Broderson, S.P., Anterior guidance—the key to successful occlusal treatment. *J Prosthet Dent*, 1978. **39**(4): p. 396–400.

 9 Schuyler, C.H., The function and importance of incisal guidance in oral rehabilitation. 1963. *J Prosthet Dent*, 2001. **86**(3): p. 219–232.

10 Mall, P., K. Singh, J. Rao, and L. Kumar, Rehabilitation of anterior teeth with customised incisal guide table. *BMJ Case Rep*, 2013. **2013**: p. bcr2013009484.

11 Hobo, S., Twin-tables technique for occlusal rehabilitation: Part I—mechanism of anterior guidance. *J Prosthet Dent*, 1991. **66**(3): p. 299–303.

12 Ogawa, T., K. Koyano, and T. Suetsugu, The influence of anterior guidance and condylar guidance on mandibular protrusive movement. *J Oral Rehabil*, 1997. **24**(4): p. 303–309.

13 Krishnamurthy, S., R.B. Hallikerimath, and P.S. Mandroli, An assessment of curve of Spee in healthy human permanent dentitions: a cross sectional analytical study in a group of young Indian population. *J Clin Diagn Res*, 2017. **11**(1): p. ZC53–ZC57.

14 Marshall, S.D., K. Kruger, R.G. Franciscus, and T.E. Southard, Development of the mandibular curve of Spee and maxillary compensating curve: a finite element model. *PLoS One*, 2019. **14**(12): p. e0221137.

15 Goyal, B.K., Bennett movement of mandible. *J Indian Dent Assoc*, 1973. **45**(12): p. 371–375.

16 Ferro, K. J. The glossary of prosthodontic terms: ninth edition. *J Prosthet Dent*, 2017. **117**: p. e1–e105.

17 Matsumura, H., Y. Tsukiyama, and K. Koyano, Analysis of sagittal condylar path inclination in consideration of Fischer's angle. *J Oral Rehabil*, 2006. **33**(7): p. 514–519.

5

Mandibular Movements

5.1 Introduction

Mandibular movement is also known as mandibular kinematics, and it has wide applications in clinical dentistry and also provides a basis for concepts of dental occlusion [1–4]. The mandibular movements are related to the envelope of motion and are traced out by the central incisor point. The mandibular movements can be studied in the various planes of the body.

Using a series of planes, the human body can be divided into three different dimensions. As shown in Figure 5.1 [5], in the human body, there are three basic planes [6].

- Sagittal plane: This plane divides the human body into left and right portions.
- Frontal (vertical) plane: A frontal, vertical, or coronal plane divides the body into posterior and anterior (dorsal and ventral) portions.
- Transverse (horizontal) plane: A transverse, horizontal, or axial plane divides the body into head and tail (cranial and caudal) portions.

The body planes have several uses within the anatomy field, including in descriptions of body motion, anatomy, embryology, medical imaging, and surgery. The mandibular movement can be seen across various planes, i.e. downward and upward movement in the frontal plane, left and right movement in the horizontal plane, and backward and forward movement in the sagittal plane.

5.2 Mandibular Movements

The temporomandibular joints (TMJs) are suspended from the skull with the help of muscles, ligaments, tendons, nerves, and vessels. With the condyles in their condylar fossae, their movement occurs in a three-dimensional (3D) space. The basic movements shown by the mandible are jaw closing and opening, elevation, depression, protrusion, retraction, and lateral movements [7].

Introduction to the Masticatory System and Dental Occlusion, First Edition. Dinesh Rokaya.
© 2025 John Wiley & Sons Ltd. Published 2025 by John Wiley & Sons Ltd.

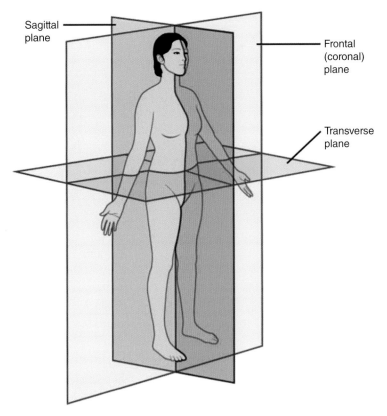

Sagittal plane

Frontal (coronal) plane

Transverse plane

Figure 5.1 Different body planes. Reference [5] / Wikimedia Commons / CC BY 4.0.

In the movement of the mandible, there are several anatomical factors that play a role.

- Condylar guidance: During a contralateral protrusive movement of the jaw, the inclined pathway traveled by the condyle.
- Incisal guidance: In a horizontal movement of the jaw along the palatal surfaces of the upper anterior teeth, the inclined pathway traveled by the mandibular anterior teeth.
- Posterior guidance: The interrelations of the posterior tooth determine it.
- Ligaments, vessels, nerves, and muscles.

Through the head of a condyle, the rotation of each TMJ takes place about an axis (Figure 5.2) [7]. The basic TMJ movements are rotation (of the condyle) and translation (of the condyle disk assembly) [7–9]. Rotation alone produces relatively little opening movement. There is a possibility for the TMJ to slide forward (protrusion) even without rotation. During mastication, there are constant combinations of rotation and translation.

Mandibular movements have been studied during speech and swallowing. For the mandibular movements during speech, it has been found that a high percentage of occlusal contacts are seen at the incisal areas [2]. This must be considered when exploring an occlusal trauma of unknown etiology. For the mandibular movements during swallowing, there is a slight contact of teeth [10] but there is no dental contact during liquid swallowing

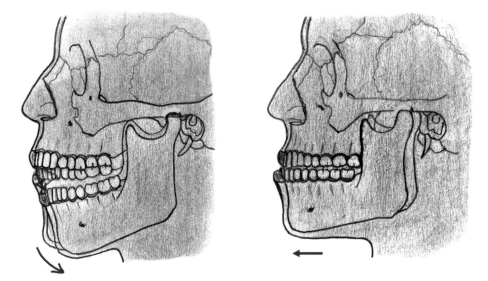

Figure 5.2 Mandibular movements showing rotational movement and translation movement. Adapted from Reference [7]; chapter published in Management of Temporomandibular Disorders and Occlusion, 7th edition, Okeson J.P., Mechanics of mandibular movements, page 63–64, Copyright Elsevier (2013).

with the aid of a straw between the lips [3]. Čimić et al. [10] studied the kinematics of the mandible and the condyles and investigated the actual movement paths and position of the mandible and condyles during the process of swallowing. They found that the average sagittal incisal point movement during swallowing was toward anterior (0.30 ± 0.53 mm) and superior (0.81 ± 0.84 mm). The mean mandibular lateral movement was 0.1 ± 0.1 mm. They mentioned that retrusion during swallowing is not compulsion but there is a slight tendency of condylar movement toward the posterior. There is a certain variation in the mandibular movements in the square mandible [11]. It is found that despite a sufficient lateral excursion, the motion of the mandible is limited by some factors at opening, suggesting the mode of lateral movements in square mandible patients.

5.2.1 Rotational Movements

Within the condyles, the rotation of condyles occurs during mouth opening and closing around the axis. The separation and then the occlusion of the teeth can be done without changing the position of the condyles. Within the inferior cavity of the TMJ joint, the rotation takes place. Rotational movement of the mandible occurs around the axis in three planes: horizontal, vertical/ frontal, and sagittal [7, 12, 13].

5.2.1.1 Horizontal Axis of Rotation

The movement of the mandible takes place in a hinge movement around the horizontal axis, i.e. the opening and closing motion, and the axis is known as the hinge axis

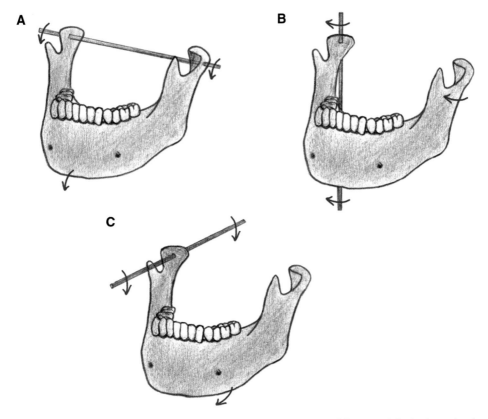

Figure 5.3 Rotational mandibular movements. A, Rotation of mandible around the horizontal axis. B, Rotation of the mandible around the vertical (frontal) axis. C, Rotation of mandible around the sagittal axis. Adapted from Reference [7]; chapter published in Management of Temporomandibular Disorders and Occlusion, 7th edition, Okeson J.P., Mechanics of mandibular movements, page 63, Copyright Elsevier (2013).

(Figure 5.3A) [7]. While the translation of the axis accompanies all other rotational movements around the axis, the hinge movement is the only movement that is purely rotational. The axis where the rotation of the mandible is purely open, occurring in the case when the condyles are in the most superior position in the articular fossae, is known as the terminal hinge axis (THA). However, it is a rarity for the rotation around the terminal hinge to occur during normal function.

5.2.1.2 Vertical Axis of Rotation

This movement occurs around the vertical axis when one (rotating) condyle moves anteriorly out of the terminal hinge position with the other (nonrotating) condyle remaining in the terminal hinge position (Figure 5.3B) [7]. This movement does occur in conjunction with the other movements. This movement does not occur alone normally due to the articular eminence's inclination causing the tilt of the vertical axis while the condyle moves anteriorly.

5.2.1.3 Sagittal Axis of Rotation

In the cases where the inferior movement of one condyle takes place, with the other remaining in the terminal hinge position, the movement of mandibles around the sagittal axis occurs (Figure 5.3C) [7]. This movement occurs in conjunction with other movements. Due to the prevention of the inferior condyle displacement because of the musculature and ligaments of the TMJ, this movement does not occur normally.

5.2.2 Translational Movements

Translation of the condyle occurs as the mandible is moved forward (Figure 5.4) [14]. Within the joint between the articular fossa's inferior surface and the articular disc's superior surface, specifically in its superior cavity, there is the translation of condyle. During

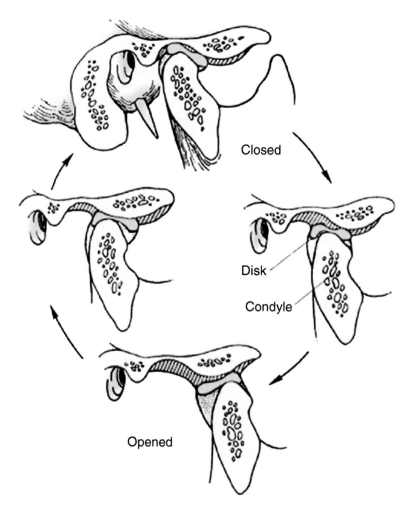

Closed

Disk

Condyle

Opened

Figure 5.4 Opening and closing of the mandible showing the relationship between the disc and condyle. Reproduced from Reference [14] / with permission from Elsevier.

most movements, both translation and rotation of condyles take place concurrently [13] while the mandibular rotation is around single or multiple axes [7].

In the sliding movement, from the mandibular fossa, the head of the mandible and disc slide together forward and downward (Figure 5.6) [14]. The axis of rotation descends to a position that is just about between the left and right foramina of the mandible from the condylar heads. The steepness of the mandibular fossa governs the intercuspation of teeth in occlusion which is the condylar guidance angle. During denture construction, in order to record the guidance angle, sliding movements are used.

5.2.2.1 Range of Movements

Normally, the rotation of the condyle shows a linear decrease or increase of around 2°/mm translation during opening or closing [15]. There is greater variation shown by closing movements in translation and rotation. It was found that there is no difference between females and males with respect to the condylar rotation but a larger maximum interincisal opening is seen in males compared to females and a greater length of the mandible in males [16]. Larger mandible results in increased mouth opening with the same degree of rotation of condyle.

5.3 Single Plane Border Movements

Moving the mandible in each reference plane through the outer range of motion within the limits is known as the border movement [7]. The movement is restricted by the articular surfaces of the TMJs, ligaments, teeth alignment, and morphology. The outer range of motion does not determine the functional movements (mastication, swallowing, and speech), and thus cannot be considered as border movements [7].

5.3.1 Sagittal Plane Border and Functional Movements

The motion of the mandible in the sagittal plane has four definite movements (Figure 5.5) as follows [7, 15]:

a) Posterior opening border movements
b) Anterior opening border movements
c) Superior contact border movements
d) Functional movements

5.3.1.1 Posterior Opening Border Movements

This movement takes place in the sagittal plane and has two stages. The initial stage is where the condyles are in the terminal hinge position; the most superior positions

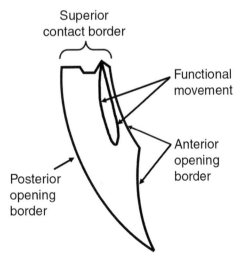

Figure 5.5 Border movements of the mandible in the sagittal plane.

A   B

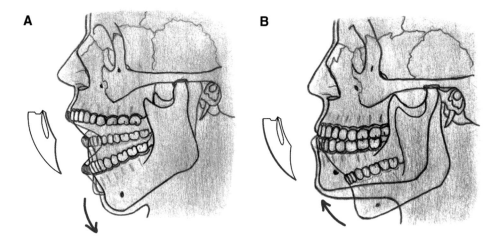

Figure 5.6 Sagittal border movement of the mandible while opening and closing. A, Rotation of the mandible during opening, showing the second stage. The condyle translates below the articular eminence while the mouth opens to the maximum. B, Anterior closing border movement of the mandible in the sagittal plane. Adapted from Reference [7]; chapter published in Management of Temporomandibular Disorders and Occlusion, 7th edition, Okeson J.P., Mechanics of mandibular movements, page 64–65, Copyright Elsevier (2013).

are in the articular fossae (Figure 5.5). From this position, centric relation (CR), i.e. movement of the hinge axis occurs. The mouth is opened in a rotation without any translation. In CR, the mandible is purely rotated to only 20–25 mm between the incisal edges of mandibular and maxillary incisors [7]. During this opening phase, there is a tightening of the TM ligaments, thereafter, opening happens in the translation of the condyles [7]. The second stage results when the mandibular axis of rotation gets shifted to the bodies of rami (Figure 5.6A) [7]. At this stage, the condyles move inferiorly and anteriorly while the mandible rotates around the horizontal axis moving through the rami. When the maximum opening (40–60 mm) is achieved, further movement is restricted by the capsular ligaments at the condyles [7].

5.3.1.2 Anterior Opening Border Movements

Following the maximum opening of the mandible, the closure with contraction of the inferior lateral pterygoid muscles causes the anterior closing border movement (Figure 5.6B) [7]. In the maximum opening, the condylar position is most anterior. While closing the mandible from the maximum opening to the maximum protruded position, a pure hinge movement can occur. The stylomandibular ligaments partly determine the maximum protrusive position and the condyles' posterior movement results from the tightening of these ligaments. It is not purely a hinge movement [7].

5.3.1.3 Superior Contact Border Movements

The superior contact border movements are determined by the occluding surfaces of the teeth: (i) the amount of discrepancy between ICP and CR, (ii) the posterior teeth's cuspal inclines' steepness, (iii) the anterior teeth's horizontal and vertical overlap amount, (iv) the maxillary anterior teeth's lingual morphology, and (v) the teeth's general inter-arch relationships [15]. There is a presence of tooth contact throughout the entirety of this movement. Generally, in the CR position, single or more opposing posterior teeth exhibit tooth contacts. The initial tooth contact CR can be seen between the distal inclines of the mandibular tooth and the mesial inclines of the maxillary tooth [7]. Furthermore, muscular force to the mandible results in a superoanterior shift from CR to the ICP. This movement is present in approximately 90% of the population which is about 1–1.25 mm in distance and may have a lateral component [17].

Mandibular movement in the horizontal direction is shown in Figure 5.7 [7]. When there is forward movement of the mandible from ICP, contact occurs between the maxillary anterior teeth's lingual incline and mandibular anterior teeth's incisal edges (Figure 5.7A) [7]. This persists until there is an edge-to-edge relation between the anterior teeth of the maxilla and mandible, during which a horizontal pathway is followed. Until the case of the mandibular teeth's incisal edges passes away from the maxillary teeth's incisal edges, the horizontal movement continues (Figure 5.7B) [7]. Until there is posterior teeth contact, the mandible shows a movement in the superior direction at this point (Figure 5.7C) [7]. The maximum protrusive movement is then controlled by the posterior teeth's occlusal surfaces, which are joined with the anterior opening border movement's most superior position (Figure 5.7D) [7].

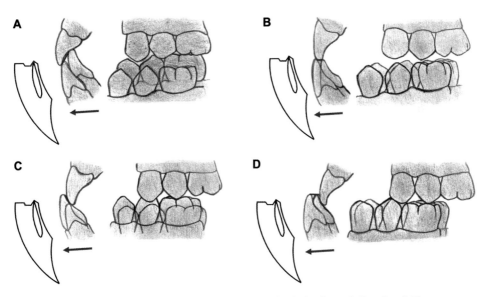

Figure 5.7 Sagittal border movement of the mandible in the horizontal direction. A, The contacts between the mandibular anterior teeth' incisal edges and maxillary anterior teeth' lingual surfaces form an inferior movement. B, The horizontal movement by the mandible as the mandibular and maxillary teeth' incisal edges pass each other. C, Continuous movement in the forward direction leads to superior movement, further leading to contact with posterior teeth. D, Until maximum protrusion, which the ligaments establish, further movement is determined by the surfaces of the posterior tooth. Adapted from Reference [7]; chapter published in Management of Temporomandibular Disorders and Occlusion, 7th edition, Okeson J.P., Mechanics of mandibular movements, page 65–66, Copyright Elsevier (2013).

When no discrepancies are present between ICP and CR, there is an alteration of the superior contact border movement's initial description. There is an absence of a superior slide from CR to ICP. There occurs an engagement of the anterior teeth due to the beginning protrusive movement and an inferior movement of the mandible takes place. The lingual anatomy of the anterior teeth of the maxilla can detect this in the situation where the condyles are in CR, there is a coinciding of the superior contact border movement with the teeth's ICP [7].

5.3.1.4 Functional Movements

Functional movements are free movements that take place when the mandible exhibits some functional activity within the border movements. ICP is required for most functional activities. The mandible is situated approximately 2–4 mm underneath the ICP when at rest [18]. A term to define this particular position is the clinical rest position. There have been suggestions from a few studies regarding its variability [19, 20]. In situations where the position of the mandible is approximately 3 mm anterior and 8 mm inferior to the ICP, the activity of the muscles of mastication is at its lowest [19]. The myotatic reflex is activated due to the function not being able to take place from this position, and this can be verified by the increased levels of electromyographic muscle activity [7, 18]. To achieve immediate function, the teeth can be brought together in this position quickly and effectively.

In the sagittal plane during the examination of chewing stroke, the beginning of the movement is seen to be in the ICP. The movement also shows a downward drop and a slight forward shift to the desired opening position (Figure 5.8) [7]. Subsequently, there is a return movement slightly posterior to the opening movement in a pathway that is straighter.

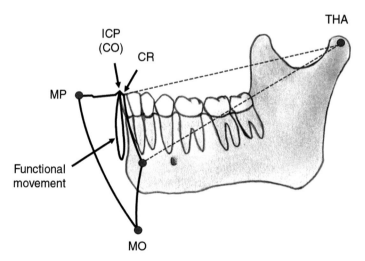

Figure 5.8 The border movements and chewing stroke in the sagittal plane. ICP = Intercuspal position, CO = Centric occlusion, CR = Centric relation, MP = Maximum protrusion, MO = Maximum opening, THA = Terminal hinge axis.

5.3.2 Horizontal Plane Border and Functional Movements

In the horizontal plane, for the recording of the movement of the mandible, there has been the use of a Gothic arch tracer [7]. There are two attachments: to the mandibular teeth, there is a recording stylus, and to the maxillary teeth, there is a recording plate. As mandibular movement is exhibited in the horizontal plane, a line is generated on the recording plate by the stylus coinciding with the movement, which helps to record the mandibular border movements. The movement is viewed as a rhomboid shape with four distinct movement components and a functional component (Figure 5.9) [7].

5.3.2.1 Right Lateral Border Movements

The mandible returns to CR and there is a recording of the right lateral border movements after there is a recording of the left border movements. An anterior, medial, and inferior movement of the left condyle is caused by the contraction of the left inferior lateral pterygoid muscle. The CR position is maintained by the right condyle if the right inferior lateral pterygoid muscle can maintain its relaxed state. As a result, a right lateral border movement (e.g. the right condyle's front axis being orbited by the left condyle) is the resulting mandibular movement. In this movement, the right condyle is the rotating condyle, and the left condyle is called the orbiting condyle. This movement generates a line on the recording plane, coinciding with the right lateral border movement (Figure 5.10A) [7].

5.3.2.2 Continued Right Lateral Border Movements with Protrusion

When the continuous contraction of the left and right inferior lateral pterygoid muscle takes place in the case where the mandible is in the right lateral border position, there is an anterior movement to the left exhibited by the right condyle. Since the maximum anterior position is already achieved by the left condyle, the mandibular midline shifts back coinciding with the midline of the maxilla due to the right condyle's movement to the maximum anterior position (Figure 5.10B) [7]. In the horizontal plane, this completes the border movement of the mandible.

5.3.2.3 Left Lateral Border Movements

When the right inferior lateral pterygoid muscles contract, there is the anterior, medial, and inferior movement of the right condyle. The relaxation of the left inferior lateral

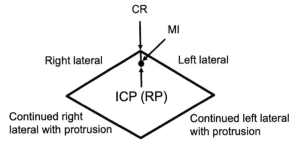

Figure 5.9 Border movements of the mandible in the horizontal plane. It consists of left lateral, continued left lateral with a protrusion, right lateral, and continued right lateral with protrusion. CR = Centric relation, ICP = Maximal intercuspal position.

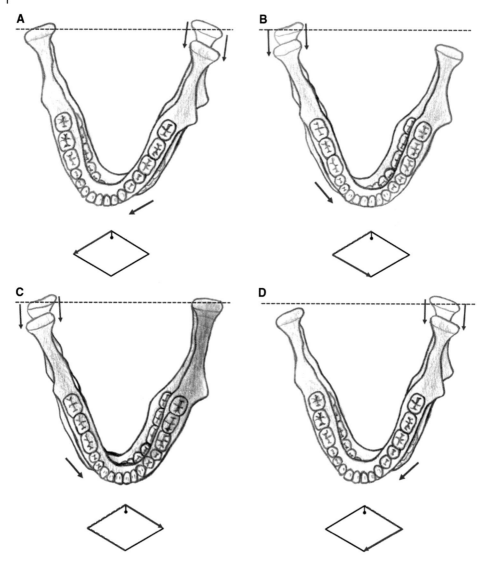

Figure 5.10 Right and left lateral border movement in the horizontal plane. A, The record of the right lateral border movement. B, The record of the continued right lateral border movement with protrusion. C, The record of the left lateral border movement. D, The record of continued left lateral border movement with protrusion. Adapted from Reference [7]; chapter published in Management of Temporomandibular Disorders and Occlusion, 7th edition, Okeson J.P., Mechanics of mandibular movements, page 68–69, Copyright Elsevier (2013).

pterygoid results in the left condyle remaining in CR; this results in a left lateral border movement (i.e. the left condyle's frontal axis being orbited around by the right condyle). Therefore, the left condyle is termed a working condyle or rotating condyle because of the rotation of the mandible around it. On the other hand, nonworking condyle or orbiting condyle is the term given to the right condyle due to its orbit being around the rotating condyle. During this movement, a line will be generated by the stylus on the recording plate coinciding with the left border movement (Figure 5.10C) [7].

5.3.2.4 Continued Left Lateral Border Movements with Protrusion

When the continuous contraction of the right inferior lateral pterygoid muscle coincides with the left inferior lateral pterygoid muscle's contraction, with the mandible being in the left lateral border position, there will be a resulting anterior movement of the left condyle to the right. Since the maximum anterior position is already achieved by the right condyle, the mandibular midline shifts back coinciding with the midline of the maxilla due to the left condyle's movement to the maximum anterior position (Figure 5.10D) [7].

There can be a generation of lateral movements diversifying the mandibular opening level. Successive smaller tracings will be obtained during the generation of border movement with an increasing degree of opening until insignificant, or no lateral movement takes place at the maximally open position [7].

5.3.2.5 Functional Movements

The functional movements generally take place close to the ICP in the horizontal plane similar to that in the sagittal plane. The jaw movement range starts in a distant manner from the maximum ICP during chewing, but the movement is closer to the ICP as there is a breakdown of the food into small particles. The existing occlusal configuration influences the mandible's exact position during chewing (Figure 5.11) [7].

5.3.3 Vertical Plane Border Movements and Functional Movements

Along with the functional component, four different movement components can be seen in a shield-shaped pattern when the motion of the mandible is observed in the frontal plane (Figure 5.12) [7]. The mandibular frontal border movements help in visualizing 3D mandibular activity.

5.3.3.1 Right Lateral Superior Border Movements

Returning of the mandible to maximum intercuspation is done once there are recordings of the movement of the left frontal border. To the right, a lateral movement is done

Figure 5.11 Functional movements in the horizontal plane. CR = Centric relation, MI = maximum intercuspation, ICP = Maximal intercuspal position, End-to-end = End-to-end position of the anterior teeth, Early area = Area in the early stages of mastication, Late area = Area in the later stages of mastication.

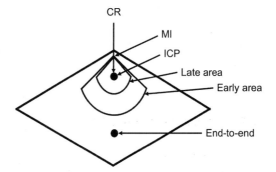

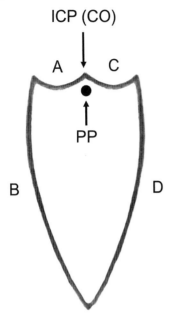

ICP (CO)

A
C

PP

B
D

Figure 5.12 Mandibular frontal border movements. A, Right lateral superior. B, Right lateral opening. C, Left lateral superior. D, Left lateral opening. CO = Centric occlusion, ICP = Maximal intercuspal position, PP = Postural position.

(Figure 5.13A), showing similarities to the left lateral superior border movement [7]. There might be minor differences due to the involved tooth contacts.

5.3.3.2 Right Lateral Opening Border Movements

A laterally convex path is produced due to the opening mandibular movement from the maximum right lateral border position showing similarities to that of the left opening movement. Ligaments produce a medially directed movement due to tightening as the maximum opening is closed, causing the shift back in the mandibular midline to the maxillary midline, thereby causing the end of the left opening movement (Figure 5.13B) [7].

5.3.3.3 Left Lateral Superior Border Movements

A movement corresponding to the lateral left is made with the mandible in ICP. There is a disclosure of a generated path that is inferiorly concave in the recording device (Figure 5.13C) [7]. The inter-arch relationships and the morphology of the mandibular and maxillary teeth which are in contact in this movement basically determine the path's precise nature. The rotating side's morphology and relationships of the condyle-disc-fossa have a secondary influence.

5.3.3.4 Left Lateral Opening Border Movements

A laterally convex path is produced due to the mandibular opening movement from the maximum left lateral superior border position. Ligaments produce a medially directed movement due to tightening as the maximum opening is done causing the shift back in the midline of the mandible to coincide with the maxillary midline (Figure 5.13D) [7].

5.3.3.5 Functional Movements

The functional movements in the frontal plane show similarities to the other planes in that ICP is the beginning and the end of the movement. Until the desired opening takes place, the mandible shows a direct inferior drop during chewing. Then, there is a shift to the side where there is the placement of the bolus and subsequently a rise. The opposing teeth break down the bolus as it approaches ICP. A quick shift to the ICP is shown by the mandible during the final millimeter of the closure (Figure 5.14) [7].

5.4 Envelope of Motion

All movements of the mandible in sagittal, vertical, and horizontal develop a 3D envelope of motion that represents the mandibular movement's maximum range that can be done from the combination of movements of the mandibular border in all three planes

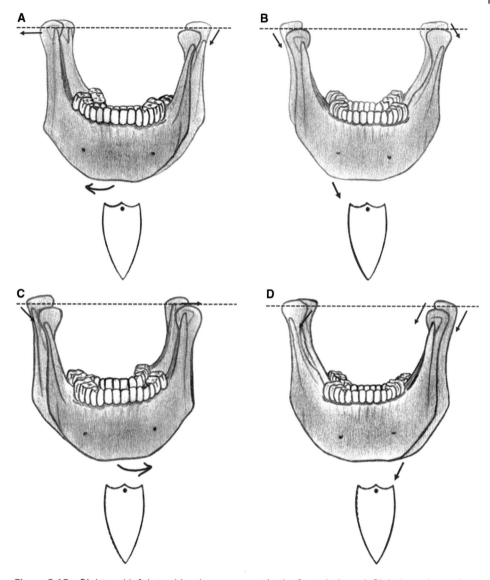

Figure 5.13 Right and left lateral border movement in the frontal plane. A, Right lateral superior border movement. B, Right lateral opening border movement. C, Left lateral superior border movement. D, Left lateral opening border movement. Adapted from Reference [7]; chapter published in Management of Temporomandibular Disorders and Occlusion, 7th edition, Okeson J.P., Mechanics of mandibular movements, page 70–71, Copyright Elsevier (2013).

(frontal, horizontal, and sagittal) [7] as shown in Figure 5.15. Despite the characteristic shape, the envelope varies depending upon the people. The tooth contacts determine the superior surface of the envelope, and the joint anatomy and ligaments determine the other borders.

To explain the mandibular movement, the right lateral excursion can be used as an example. The left condyle is forced out of its CR position as there is a contraction of musculature as well as a right mandibular movement. The anterior orbiting of the left condyle around

ICP (CO)

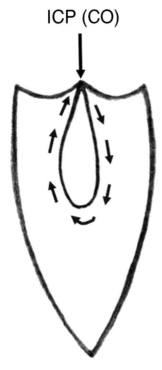

Figure 5.14 Functional movement within the mandibular border movement in the frontal plane. CO = Centric occlusion, ICP = Intercuspal position.

the right condyle's frontal axis results in it facing the articular eminence's posterior slope. Due to this, around the sagittal axis, an inferior movement of the condyle is caused, which results in the frontal axis tilt. In addition, compared to the posterior part of the mandible, a greater inferior movement in the anterior part is produced due to the contact of the anterior teeth resulting in an opening around the horizontal axis. There is an anterior and inferior shift in the horizontal axis since there is anterior and inferior movement exhibited by the left condyle [13].

This example describes a simple lateral movement, each axis simultaneously tilting for the accommodation of the movements taking place around the other axis after motion occurring around each axis (horizontal, vertical, and sagittal). This takes place within the envelope of motion, and it is under the control of the neuromuscular system.

5.5 Mandibular Movements in Diseases and Defects

The mandibular movements during functions can be affected by certain diseases and defects such as obstructive sleep apnea, bruxism, arthritis, temporomandibular disorders (TMD), and mandibulectomy [21–26].

Figure 5.15 3D envelope of motion of mandibular movement.

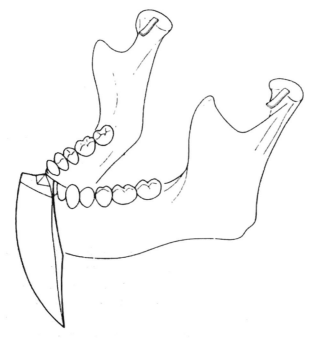

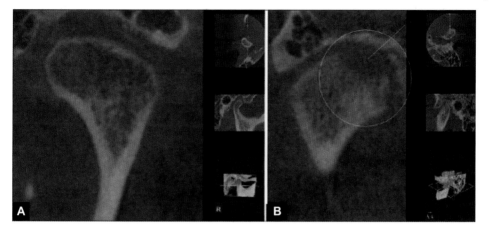

Figure 5.16 Temporomandibular joint in rheumatoid arthritis. A, Right side shows a decrease in the joint space. B, Left side shows a narrowing of the articular space and erosions on the superior head of the condyle. Reproduced from [26] / with permission of Wolters Kluwer Health, Inc.

TMD may cause changes in mandibular movements due to joint and muscular conditions [21, 27–30]. It was found that the presence of TMD shows a reduction in mandibular opening and retrusion ranges and unilateral deviation is seen during speech [21]. Celic et al. [28] found that there is a difference in the range of mandibular movements in patients with TMD in this young male population. In rheumatoid arthritis, a decrease and erosion of the joint space and narrowing of the articular space can be seen, which affects the mandibular movements [26, 31–33] as shown in Figure 5.16 [26]. Similarly, Pepin et al. [22] studied whether the sleep mandibular movements signal recorded with a triaxial gyroscopic chin sensor in patients with suspected obstructive sleep apnea. They found that in obstructive sleep apnea patients, mandibular movement signals facilitated the measurement of specific levels of respiratory effort associated with obstructive, central, or mixed apneas and/or hypopneas (Figure 5.17) [22]. A high degree of similarity was observed with the esophageal pressure gold standard signal.

In mandibulectomy patients without surgical reconstruction, the remaining mandibular segment is unstable and often deviated and, in such cases, the mastication, deglutition, and speech are affected. Takahashi et al. [23] studied the differences in mandibular movements in the sagittal, frontal, and horizontal planes for oral functions in mandibulectomy patients with and without mandibular continuity. Group I consisted of mandibulectomy without mandibular continuity and group II consisted of mandibular continuity. The findings were as follows: In group I, the border movements at the incisor showed an irregular and asymmetric envelope deviated to the resected side in the frontal plane, whereas group II showed a smooth and symmetric envelope. In group I, the rotational angles during border movements and mastication (in the frontal plane), during speech (in all planes), and during deglutition (in the frontal and horizontal plane), were significantly larger compared to group II. The border and all functional movements in mandibulectomy patients showed characteristic movements in the rotation of the mandible in the frontal plane, which is a useful parameter for the assessment of mandibular movements in mandibulectomy patients.

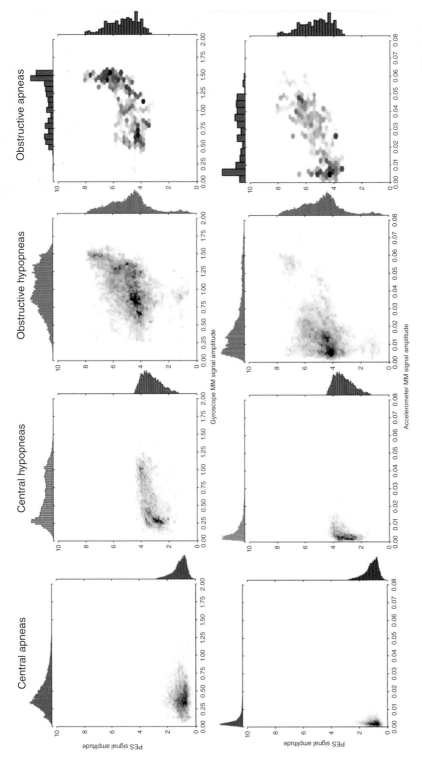

Figure 5.17 Joint distribution and esophageal pressure and mandibular movement amplitudes for sleep apnea. Reproduced from Reference [22] / with permission from Taylor & Francis group.

References

1 Brown, T., Mandibular movements. *Monogr Oral Sci*, 1975. **4**: p. 126–150.
2 Peraire, M., J. Salsench, J. Torrent, J. Nogueras, and J. Samso, Study of mandibular movements during speech. *Cranio*, 1990. **8**(4): p. 324–331.
3 Nogueras, J., J. Salsench, J. Torrent, J. Samsó, M. Peraire, and J.M. Anglada, Study of the mandibular movements during swallowing. *Cranio*, 1991. **9**(4): p. 322–327.
4 Pound, E., The mandibular movements of speech and their seven related values. *J Prosthet Dent*, 1966. **16**(5): p. 835–843.
5 *Wikimedia Commons*. Planes of Body. https://commons.wikimedia.org *(Accessed on November 28, 2023)*. 2023.
6 Kim, E.S., T. Kim, and J.-W. Kim, Three-dimensional modelling of a humanoid in three planes and a motion scheme of biped turning in standing. *IET Control Theory A*, 2009. **3**: p. 1155–1166.
7 Okeson, J.P., *Management of Temporomandibular Disorders and Occlusion*. 7th ed. 2013, St. Louis, Missouri: Mosby.
8 *The temporomandibular joints, muscles of mastication, and the infratemporal and pterygopalatine fossae*. 2020; Available from: https://pocketdentistry.com/24-the-temporomandibular-joints-muscles-of-mastication-and-the-infratemporal-and-pterygopalatine-fossae/ (Accessed on November 28, 2023).
9 Eriksson, P.O., B. Häggman-Henrikson, E. Nordh, and H. Zafar, Co-ordinated mandibular and head-neck movements during rhythmic jaw activities in man. *J Dent Res*, 2000. **79**(6): p. 1378–1384.
10 Čimić, S., S.K. Šimunković, R.K. Gospić, T. Badel, N. Dulčić, and A. Ćatić, Movements of temporomandibular condyles during swallowing. *Coll Antropol*, 2015. **39**(1): p. 159–164.
11 Hirai, S., T. Ogawa, Y. Shigeta, E. Ando, R. Hirabayashi, T. Ikawa, S. Kasama, S. Fukushima, and Y. Matsuka, Characteristics of mandibular movements in patients with square mandible. *Oral Surg Oral Med Oral Pathol Oral Radiol Endod*, 2009. **108**(5): p. e75–81.
12 Mapelli, A., D. Galante, N. Lovecchio, C. Sforza, and V.F. Ferrario, Translation and rotation movements of the mandible during mouth opening and closing. *Clin Anat*, 2009. **22**(3): p. 311–318.
13 Lindauer, S.J., G. Sabol, R.J. Isaacson, and M. Davidovitch, Condylar movement and mandibular rotation during jaw opening. *Am J Orthod Dentofacial Orthop*, 1995. **107**(6): p. 573–577.
14 Howard, J.A., Temporomandibular joint disorders in children. *Dent Clin North Am*, 2013. **57**(1): p. 99–127.
15 Salaorni, C. and S. Palla, Condylar rotation and anterior translation in healthy human temporomandibular joints. *Schweiz Monatsschr Zahnmed*, 1994. **104**: p. 415–422.
16 Naeije, M., Local kinematic and anthropometric factors related to the maximum mouth opening in healthy individuals. *J Oral Rehabil*, 2002. **29**: p. 534–539.
17 Posselt, U., Movement areas of the mandible. *J Prosthet Dent*, 1957. **7**: p. 375–385.
18 Garnick, J. and S.P. Ramfjord, An electromyographic and clinical investigation. *J Prosthet Dent*, 1962. **12**: p. 895–911.

19 Rugh, J.D. and C.J. Drago, Vertical dimension: a study of clinical rest position and jaw muscle activity. *J Prosthet Dent*, 1981. **45**: p. 670–675.

20 Atwood, D.A., A critique of reseach of the rest position of the mandible. *J Prosthet Dent*, 1966. **16**: p. 848–854.

21 Bianchini, E.M., G. Paiva, and C.R. de Andrade, Mandibular movement patterns during speech in subjects with temporomandibular disorders and in asymptomatic individuals. *Cranio*, 2008. **26**(1): p. 50–58.

22 Pepin, J.L., N.N. Le-Dong, V. Cuthbert, N. Coumans, R. Tamisier, A. Malhotra, and J.B. Martinot, Mandibular movements are a reliable noninvasive alternative to esophageal pressure for measuring respiratory effort in patients with sleep apnea syndrome. *Nat Sci Sleep*, 2022. **14**: p. 635–644.

23 Takahashi, M., M. Hideshima, I. Park, H. Taniguchi, and T. Ohyama, Study of mandibular movements in mandibulectomy patients—border movements and functional movements during mastication, deglutition and speech. *J Med Dent Sci*, 1999. **46**(2): p. 93–103.

24 Kjellberg, H., Juvenile chronic arthritis: dentofacial morphology, growth, mandibular function and orthodontic treatment. *Swed Dent J Suppl*, 1995. **109**: p. 1–56.

25 Barbosa Tde, S., L.S. Miyakoda, L. Pocztaruk Rde, C.P. Rocha, and M.B. Gavião, Temporomandibular disorders and bruxism in childhood and adolescence: review of the literature. *Int J Pediatr Otorhinolaryngol*, 2008. **72**(3): p. 299–314.

26 Sodhi, A., S. Naik, A. Pai, and A. Anuradha, Rheumatoid arthritis affecting temporomandibular joint. *Contemp Clin Dent*, 2015. **6**(1): p. 124–127.

27 Celić, R., V. Jerolimov, D. Knezović Zlatarić, and B. Klaić, Measurement of mandibular movements in patients with temporomandibular disorders and in asymptomatic subjects. *Coll Antropol*, 2003. **27** Suppl 2: p. 43–49.

28 Celic, R., V. Jerolimov, and K.Z. Dubravka, Relationship of slightly limited mandibular movements to temporomandibular disorders. *Braz Dent J*, 2004. **15**(2): p. 151–154.

29 Bonjardim, L.R., M.B. Gavião, L.J. Pereira, and P.M. Castelo, Mandibular movements in children with and without signs and symptoms of temporomandibular disorders. *J Appl Oral Sci*, 2004. **12**(1): p. 39–44.

30 Cortese, S.G., L.M. Oliver, and A.M. Biondi, Determination of range of mandibular movements in children without temporomandibular disorders. *Cranio*, 2007. **25**(3): p. 200–205.

31 Delantoni, A., E. Spyropoulou, J. Chatzigiannis, and P. Papademitriou, Sole radiographic expression of rheumatoid arthritis in the temporomandibular joints: a case report. *Oral Surg Oral Med Oral Pathol Oral Radiol Endod*, 2006. **102**(4): p. e37–e40.

32 Goupille, P., B. Fouquet, P. Cotty, D. Goga, and J.P. Valat, Direct coronal computed tomography of the temporomandibular joint in patients with rheumatoid arthritis. *Br J Radiol*, 1992. **65**(779): p. 955–960.

33 O'Connor, R.C., F. Fawthrop, R. Salha, and A.J. Sidebottom, Management of the temporomandibular joint in inflammatory arthritis: involvement of surgical procedures. *Eur J Rheumatol*, 2017. **4**(2): p. 151–156.

6

Mastication, Swallowing, and Speech

6.1   Introduction

The three major functions of the masticatory system are mastication, swallowing, and speech. Expression of emotions and respiration are assisted by secondary functions. All the functional motions are extremely well-coordinated, complex, neuromuscular events. To achieve a desired function, the sensory input from the anatomic structures of the masticatory system (i.e. cheeks, lips, teeth, periodontal ligaments, tongue, and palate) is obtained and merged in the central pattern generator (CPG) with existing reflex activity and acquired muscle engrams. In the function of the masticatory system, teeth occlusion plays a vital role, so it is necessary to understand the mechanism of these significant functional activities.

6.2   Mastication

Mastication involves chewing food by maxillary and mandibular teeth for swallowing and digestion [1]. It is pleasurable and enjoyable as it utilizes the senses of touch, taste, and smell [2]. The feedback mechanism retards these positive feelings when the stomach is quite full. Mastication itself is a function that is complex, as it not only utilizes the supportive periodontal structures, muscles, and teeth but also other oral and facial structures such as the palate, salivary glands, lips, tongue, and cheeks [2]. This functional activity is usually automatic and pragmatically involuntary. However, one can willingly bring it under voluntary control when desired. Mastication is important not only for intake the of food but also for the mental, systemic, and physical functions of the body [3]. Masticatory muscle function also has an influence on craniofacial growth along with the maxilla and mandible [4–6]. The masticatory muscle hyperfunction leads to increased sutural growth and bone apposition, resulting, in turn, in the growth of the maxilla and the dental arches. Furthermore, an increase in the function of the masticatory muscles leads to the growth of the mandible with angular, coronoid, and condylar processes [5]. Mastication or chewing is also an efficient stress-coping behavior [7]. It has been shown that chewing gum during stress can decrease plasma and salivary cortisol levels and can reduce mental stress [7–9].

Introduction to the Masticatory System and Dental Occlusion, First Edition. Dinesh Rokaya.
© 2025 John Wiley & Sons Ltd. Published 2025 by John Wiley & Sons Ltd.

6.2.1 Masticatory Mechanism and Chewing Stroke

The process of mastication is a periodic and well-controlled union and disunion of mandibular and maxillary teeth. CGP controls this activity. CGP is a group of neurons inside the brainstem that controls rhythmic muscle movements like chewing, breathing, and walking [10, 11]. Chewing stroke is represented by each closing and opening movement of the mandible and can be classified into a closing phase and an opening phase, respectively. The closing movement of the mandible is subclassified into crushing and grinding phases.

6.2.2 Incision of Food

On the introduction of food into the mouth, the mandible lowers down due to the primary action of the depressor muscles. The next step is the incision of the food. Bilateral, simultaneous, and synchronous contraction and relaxation of masticatory muscles occur, which include contraction of the masseters (deep layer assisted by the superficial layers), contraction of the temporalis (medial and posterior bundles assisted by anterior bundles), and contraction of the lateral pterygoid (superior head assisted by the inferior heads). These actions elevate and protract the mandible producing incision of food by the incisors.

6.2.3 Crushing and Grinding of Food

With the reduction of food, the more specialized cycle of mastication begins. While chewing the food, the mastication cycle continues with depression and elevation of the mandible in a configuration of a teardrop.

6.2.4 Masticatory Cycle

Mastication involves the incision of food and crushing of the food followed by a masticatory cycle which consists of four phases: opening, closing, occlusion, and exit. This cycle starts with the lowering of the mandible and the involvement of muscle fibers. During mastication, the condylar movements involve circular paths for both balancing and working condyles. The balancing side translations are more extensive than the working side. This movement results in a teardrop-shaped configuration of the complete chewing stroke (Figure 6.1) [2]. The apex of the teardrop is the level of the opposing teeth during occlusion.

Homogenous chewing strokes are performed again and again as the food gets fragmented during mastication. The following sequence occurs during a solo chewing stroke in the frontal plane.

The first phase or crushing phase of closure is characterized by the trapping of food in between the teeth. As there is a close approximation of teeth, lateral displacement is decreased such that when there is a distance of 3 mm between the teeth, the jaw occupies a place just 3–4 mm lateral to the initial chewing stroke position [2]. The cheek and tongue muscles play a vital role during mastication. The lips direct and control the intake when the food is brought into the mouth, while also closing the oral cavity. Especially during liquid consumption, lips play a vital role. The major role of the tongue is not only in taste perception but also involves adequate chewing by maneuvering food

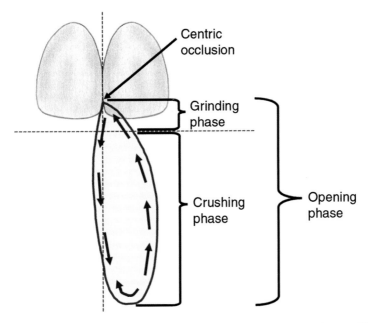

Figure 6.1 Frontal view of the chewing stroke. Adapted from Reference [2]; chapter published in Management of Temporomandibular Disorders and Occlusion, 7th edition, Okeson J.P., Functional Neuroanatomy and Physiology of the Masticatory System, page 31, Copyright Elsevier (2013).

inside the oral cavity. The tongue shifts the semicrushed food in between the teeth in another chewing stroke of the opening phase for its additional breakdown. As the tongue repositions the food, side by side the cheek, comprising the buccinator muscle, completes the same work as the buccal part. The masticatory cycle involves following steps after the incision.

a) Phase 1: Opening
b) Phase 2: Closing
c) Phase 3: Occlusion
d) Phase 4: Exit

6.2.4.1 Phase 1: Opening

In this phase, the mandible sets down from the occlusion to the point where the interincisal part is separated by 16–18 mm, and as the closing movement starts, it shifts laterally by 5–6 mm from the midline [2].

The condyle moves forward due to the predominant bilateral contraction of the lateral pterygoid muscle and forward translation of the disc occurs due to assisted activity of the lateral pterygoid muscle. The medial and lateral pterygoid muscles on the chewing side initially produce a greater contraction, moving the condyle forward and medially. The accessory muscles that aid in mastication are the suprahyoid and the digastric muscles which are active in lowering the mandible.

6.2.4.2 Phase 2: Closing

The mandible moves up and laterally to the chewing side in this phase. During this movement, muscles on both sides of the jaw are active. The mandibular movement to the chewing side is assisted by the medial pterygoid on the nonchewing side. Simultaneously, towards the chewing side, the masseter (superficial layer) and the temporalis (anterior bundles), assisted by the masseter (deep layer), temporalis (intermediate and posterior bundles), lateral pterygoid (superior head), and medial pterygoid, help in mandibular elevation.

6.2.4.3 Phase 3: Occlusion

This phase occurs with the maximal masticatory muscle force on the chewing side of the mandible Figure 6.2 [2]. The occlusal table of the teeth is mostly involved in this process. The food bolus is confined in between the teeth as the mandible keeps on closing which starts the grinding phase.

The neuromuscular network is permanently active during this phase. It consists of the periodontal membrane, TMJ (temporomandibular joint) capsule receptors, TMJ mechanoreceptors, vascular supply, limbic system, brain stem, and central nervous system (CNS).

Figure 6.2 also shows the muscles that participate in the process of mastication [2]. During the occlusal masticatory phase, the strong action of the masseter (superficial and deep) and medial pterygoid assisted by the temporalis muscle on the chewing side promotes the grinding of food on the chewing side. The working condyle in this phase produces limited movements while the action of the lateral pterygoid generates condylar rotation and stabilization of the disc.

The mandible is led back into the intercuspal position by the occlusal surfaces of teeth during the grinding phase. This results in the crossing of cuspal inclines of teeth past each other, allowing grinding and shearing of the food bolus. In this phase, mostly the

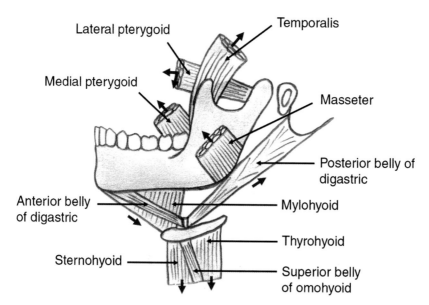

Figure 6.2 Muscles involved in the mastication.

group function predominates, and opposing occlusal surfaces come in contact during the mastication with the involvement of the cuspal inclines. If there is canine guidance, axial masticatory loads predominate at the depth of the opposing fosse.

6.2.4.4 Phase 4: Exit

With the crushing stage of mastication, the mandible moves down medially to clear away from the occlusal table of the opposing arch. Active action of the medial pterygoid and lateral pterygoid muscle (both heads) on the chewing side moves the mandible medially. This movement, to control the speed of motion, is assisted by the masseter (superficial layers) and temporalis (anterior and intermediate bundles) on the chewing side of the mandible. After this phase, a new cycle starts.

6.2.5 Mandibular Movements During Crushing and Grinding

During a normal chewing stroke while opening, there is a slight anterior movement of the mandible seen in the sagittal plane (Figure 6.3) [2, 12]. It accompanies the posterior path to some degree during the closing phase and ends up back to the centric occlusion in an anterior movement. The masticatory stage and pattern of contact of the anterior teeth determine the proportion of anterior movement [13]. Food incising is usually important during the early stages. Based on the position and alignment of the opposing incisors, there is a forward movement of the mandible for a remarkable distance during incising. The forward movement is reduced after the food is incised and introduced into the mouth. The crushed food mass is concentrated towards the posterior teeth and there occurs less anterior movement in further stages of mastication; however, the closing phase is posterior to the opening phase [12, 14].

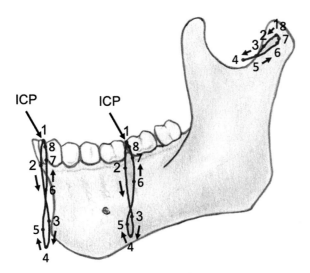

Figure 6.3 Sagittal plane of the working side indicating the chewing stroke. IP = Intercuspal position. Adapted from Reference [2]; chapter published in Management of Temporomandibular Disorders and Occlusion, 7th edition, Okeson J.P., Functional Neuroanatomy and Physiology of the Masticatory System, page 31, Copyright Elsevier (2013).

During a normal chewing stroke, the motion of the mandibular first molar differs based on the side where an individual chews, in regard to the sagittal plane. When there is movement of the mandible to the right side, the first molar of the right side moves in the direction of the incisor. To put it another way, there is a slight anterior movement of the molar during the opening phase, and it closes faintly on the posterior pathway, going anteriorly in the course of final closure when the teeth occlude.

Towards the right side, the condyle follows the same pathway, closing in a posterior position accompanied by anterior movement into the intercuspation (Figure 6.3). [2, 12, 14] If the first molar happens to be towards the opposite side, then this case shall seem to navigate from a varied pattern. On the mandible movement to the right side, a vertical drop is seen in the left mandibular first molar. Unless there is a proper completion of the opening phase, the vertical drop continues with slight anterior or posterior movement. When there is closure, a slight anterior movement is seen in the mandible and the tooth retrieves back directly to intercuspation (Figure 6.4) [2, 12].

Towards the left, the condyle goes through a similar path to that taken by the molar. In the end, no anterior movement towards the intercuspal position, either the molar or the condyle pathway, is noticed [12, 14].

Like anterior movement, the times of the mandible's lateral movement relate to the stage of mastication. At the moment when food is put into the mouth, lateral movement is higher, but this rate decreases while the food is finely broken. The quantity of lateral movement corresponds to food consistency. If the food is hard, additional lateral closure stroke becomes a high necessity before swallowing starts [12, 14].

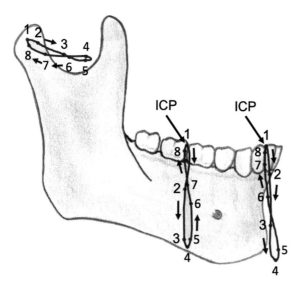

Figure 6.4 Sagittal plane of the nonworking side showing the chewing stroke. IP, Intercuspal position. Adapted from Reference [2]; chapter published in Management of Temporomandibular Disorders and Occlusion, 7th edition, Okeson J.P., Functional Neuroanatomy and Physiology of the Masticatory System, page 32, Copyright Elsevier (2013).

6.2.6   Chewing Side Preference

Although mastication can occur bilaterally, it was found that 78% of the study sample preferred side to do most of their chewing [15] with the highest number of tooth contacts in the course of the lateral glide [16]. The ones who do not have a particular preference side alter from one side to the other while chewing. When only one side of chewing is practiced, there occurs an unbalanced loading of the TMJs [17, 18]. The muscle activity patterns are preferably created to manage the magnitude and position of occlusal forces rather than TMJ forces. If the conditions are normal, such practice does not result in any issues owing to the balancing effect on the discs by superior lateral pterygoid muscles.

6.2.7   Contacts of Tooth During Mastication

During the process of mastication, it is known that there is no actual contact between the teeth [19]. According to predictions, such contact is prohibited by the food present between the teeth and acute feedback of the neuromuscular system. Immediately upon the intro-duction of food into the mouth, only little contact occurs.

When the food bolus is broken down, the contact frequency of the tooth rises. Towards the last stages of mastication, and just before swallowing, contact occurs repeatedly but there are minimum forces to the teeth [20]. Generally, two types of contacts occur, gliding and single. Gliding happens when the cuspal inclines cross through one another during the grinding and opening phases of mastication, and the single happens in the position of maximum intercuspation [21]. The majority of gliding contact (60%) occurs during chew-ing in the grinding phase and 56% in the opening phase [22]. During mastication, the mean time length for contact with a tooth was found to be 194 milliseconds.

The tooth contact continually returns sensory information to the CNS regarding the chewing stroke's character [2]. Through this feedback mechanism, modification of chew-ing stroke is permitted to the food that is being chewed. Usually, tall cusps and deep fossae encourage a highly dominant vertical chewing stroke. On the other hand, flattened or worn teeth promote chewing strokes that are broader in nature.

There are marked differences in the chewing strokes of a normal person and a person with TMJ pain [23]. Much rounded, repeated, and definite bordered chewing strokes are observed in normal individuals. In TMJ pain patients, the chewing strokes are irregular, less repeated pattern, and much shorter and slower, which is because of the pain due to the altered condylar functional movement.

6.2.8   Mastication Force

During mastication, occlusal forces are generated by the masticatory muscles and are transferred to the teeth, the enamel being the tissue that receives directly these loads [24]. The mastication force or bite force basically arises from the activity of the elevator muscles of the jaw, and it is adjusted by the craniomandibular biomechanics [25]. The force put on teeth during mastication differs from one person to another. It is often known that the force with which women can bite is lesser than men. The biting force being more in men increases with age [26, 27]. There is a report regarding the biting load range for men and women being 118–142 lbs (53.6–64.4 kg) and 79–99 lbs (35.8–44.9 kg), respectively [28]. The reported maximum biting force is 975 lbs (443 kg) [29]. The maximal force put on molars is generally several times more than on incisors. The maximum amount of force applied to the first molar is much more than that applied to the central incisors: ranging from 91 to 198 lbs (41.3–89.8 kg) at the molars and 29–51 lbs (13.2–23.1 kg) at the central incisors [30]. The maximal mastication force value of the incisor, premolar, and first molar of all the men was 43.3, 99.11, and 120.66 kg, respectively [26]. Also, with exercise and practice, individuals can raise their maximal biting force over time [22, 31]. So, an individual who consumes a greater percentage of a diet containing hard solid foods develops a powerful biting force and the action of chewing mainly happens in the premolar and first molar areas [32]. In subjects with complete dentures, the biting force is merely 1/4th of the subjects present with natural teeth. In cleft lip and palate with posterior crossbites, increased vertical overlap, and increased overjet, the temporalis muscle activity is affected [33].

The horizontal and lateral occlusion forces (Figure 6.5A) present during the functional chewing process are harmful [24, 34, 35]. These harmful forces can lead to the damage of tooth structure which is known as abfraction (Figure 6.5B) [24] and these forces can also lead to the failure of the restorations. Hence, when planning the adequate materials, and mechanical design of prostheses, implants, and treatment, careful considerations need to be made.

Hernández-Vázquez et al. [24] studied the reactions of the dental organs to the different forces occurring during chewing using a finite element model of the lower first molar and two simulations; one considered the contact between the enamel and the dentin, and the other did not take it into account. The results of the displacements for each of the axes, in the simulations with and without contact for the load of $150\,N/mm^2$, there were significant differences between the simulations that consider contact and those that do not as shown in Figure 6.6 [24].

The masticatory function is regulated by the CNS, which is the primary element to guide the functioning of mastication organ muscles. Kijak et al. [36] made an attempt to mathematically describe the mastication organ muscle functioning, taking into consideration the impact on the CNS. Figure 6.7A shows the distribution of active forces operating on the mandible and points describing its geometric structure. Figure 6.7B shows the muscles of mastication during the closing of the mandible of normal craniofacial morphology while loading the mandibular arch in the area of incisors and oof molars. Hence, the identification of muscle forces considering the impact of the nervous system can help to reflect the conditions of mastication organ muscle functioning.

6.3 Swallowing

Swallowing or deglutition is a sequence of muscular contractions that are coordinated, where the food bolus is passed from the oral cavity into the stomach by way of the esophagus. It involves reflex, and involuntary and voluntary activities of nerves and muscles [37]. The oral cavity is sealed, led by the closure of lips during the process of swallowing. The mandible is stabilized after the teeth acquire the maximal intercuspal position. Deglutition

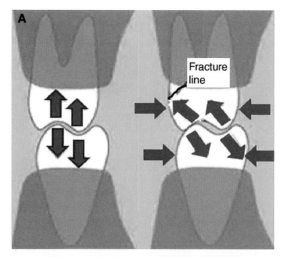

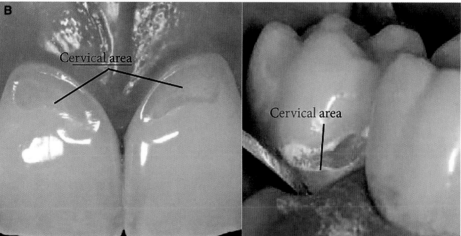

Figure 6.5 Horizontal and lateral occlusal forces on teeth and their effects on tooth structures. A, Normal and parafunctional forces acting during mastication. B, Damage to the tooth structures from the horizontal and lateral forces. Reference [24] / John Wiley & Sons / CC BY 4.0.

is dependent on various factors such as the level of food fineness, its taste, and the amount of bolus lubrication [2]. During the process of swallowing, correct movement of the hyoid bone is necessary. This movement is controlled only when the mandible is stable so that infrahyoid and suprahyoid muscles can contract.

The anatomy of the neck region of infants is different from that of adults. In the infant, teeth are not erupted, the hard palate is flatter, the larynx and hyoid bone is higher, and the epiglottis touches the back of the soft palate (Figure 6.8A) [37]. With development, the anatomy of the pharynx in humans changes. The larynx descends lower than the contact of the soft palate and epiglottis is lost, and the pharynx becomes longer vertically (Figure 6.8B) [37]. In infantile swallowing, the mandible is supported by positioning the tongue forward and in the middle of the gum pads or dental arches [38, 39].

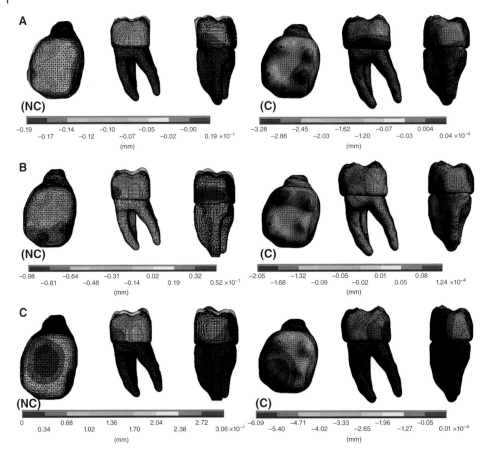

Figure 6.6 Displacement in different axes. A, X-axis. B, Y-axis. C, Z-axis. NC = Noncontact, C = Contact. Reference [24] / John Wiley & Sons / CC BY 4.0.

The adult swallow makes use of the teeth for the stability of the mandible [40]. When there is an eruption of posterior teeth into the occlusion, the mandible is braced by the occluding teeth, and the adult swallow is presumed. Even though the process of swallowing is one continual action, for analysis, it is classified into three stages here (Figure 6.9) [2].

6.3.1 First Stage

It is the voluntary stage of swallowing that initiates with the splitting of the chewed food into a bolus. This activity is mainly done by the tongue. Food bolus or mass is kept on the tongue and gently pressed in opposition to the hard palate. During this time, the tongue tip lies on the hard palate behind the incisors (Figure 6.9). The teeth are brought into contact while the lips are closed. A reflex starts off when the food bolus is present near the palatal mucosa, which creates a series of contractions in the tongue that eventually pushes the mass backward. This mass is conveyed to the pharynx after it reaches the most posterior part of the tongue [27].

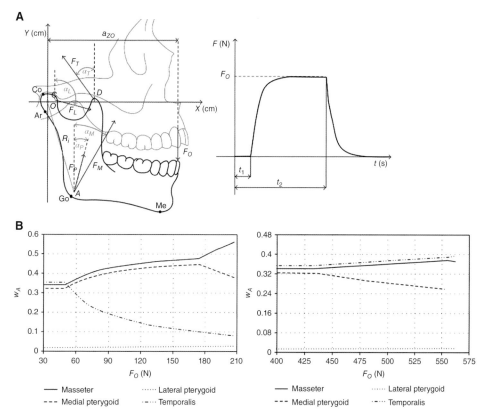

Figure 6.7 Active forces and muscles of mastication. A, Distribution of active forces operating on the mandible and points describing its geometric structure. B, Muscles of mastication during the closing of the mandible of normal craniofacial morphology during loading the mandibular arch in the area of incisors (left) and oof molars (right). Reference [36] / John Wiley & Sons / CC BY 3.0.

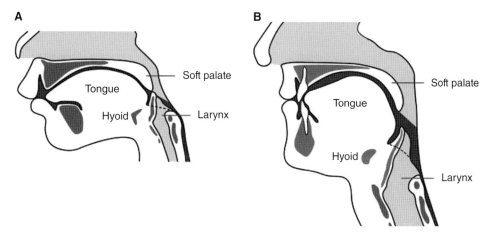

Figure 6.8 Anatomy of the orofacial and neck region. A, Infant. B, Adult. Reproduced from Reference [37] / with permission from Elsevier.

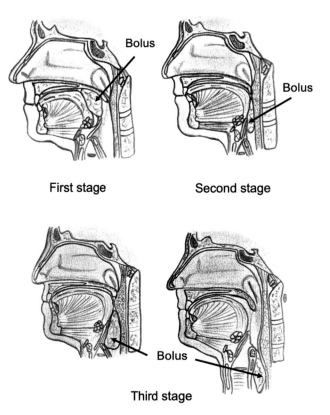

Figure 6.9 Stages of swallowing. Adapted from Reference [2]; chapter published in Management of Temporomandibular Disorders and Occlusion, 7th edition, Okeson J.P., Functional Neuroanatomy and Physiology of the Masticatory System, page 35, Copyright Elsevier (2013).

6.3.2   Second Stage

The contraction of pharyngeal constrictor muscles occurs in the pharynx when the food bolus arrives. This generates a peristaltic wave which helps to transfer the food bolus to the esophagus. The nasal passage is sealed off when the posterior pharyngeal wall is touched by the elevated soft palate. While keeping the food mass in the esophagus, the pharyngeal airway towards the trachea is blocked by epiglottis. The pharyngeal orifices associated with the eustachian tubes are opened by the muscular activity of the pharynx in this stage [2]. It is approximated that the first and second stages of swallowing all together exist for about one second.

6.3.3   Third Stage

This stage comprises advancing the food bolus from the esophagus into the stomach. To transport the bolus via the esophagus, the peristaltic waves take around six to seven seconds. When the bolus advances towards the cardiac sphincter, it gets into the stomach after the sphincter is relaxed. The muscles in the upper parts of the esophagus are mostly

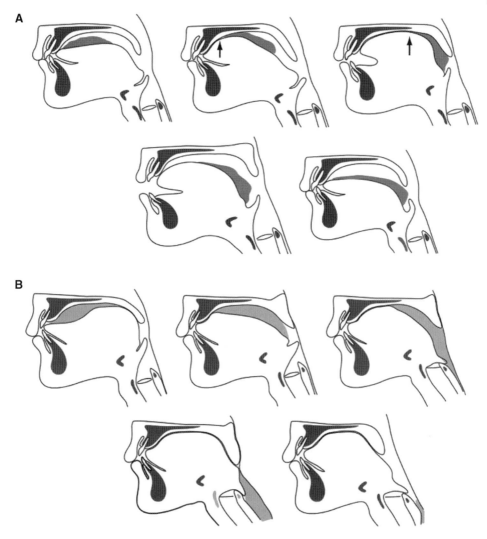

Figure 6.10 Videofluroscopy images of swallowing a solid bolus and liquid bolus. A, Swallowing a solid bolus. B, Swallowing a liquid bolus. Reproduced from Reference [37] / with permission from Elsevier.

voluntary. For additional complete mastication, these muscles may be utilized to bring back the food to the mouth, if needed. The muscles in the lower parts of the esophagus are completely involuntary [2].

There is a difference in the process of swallowing solid bolus and drinking liquid (liquid bolus) (Figure 6.10) [37]. During eating and swallowing of solid bolus, the movement of the tongue and soft palate occurs in a cyclic process with jaw movement causing open communication between the pharynx and oral cavity with no sealing of the posterior oral cavity [37, 41, 42]. In the meantime, the tongue helps the food's aroma to pass the nasal cavity through the pharynx, delivering the chemoreceptors in the nose [43–45]. During drinking, the posterior oral cavity is sealed by tongue–palate contact during the oral preparatory

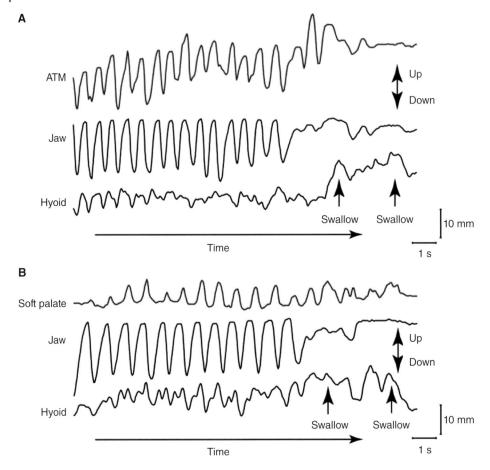

Figure 6.11 Cyclic movement of the jaw in processing is tightly coordinated with the movements of the tongue, cheek, soft palate, and hyoid bone during swallowing. Adapted from Reference [37]. A, Movements of the tongue, jaw, and hyoid bone over time. B, Movement of soft palate, jaw, and hyoid bone over time. ATM = Anterior tongue marker.

stage when the bolus is held in the oral cavity [37]. There is a cyclic movement of the jaw in processing that is coordinated with the movements of the tongue, cheek, soft palate, and hyoid bone during swallowing (Figure 6.11) [37]. It shows that the rhythmic movement of the tongue and soft palate is linked to cyclic jaw movement. The hyoid bone also moves rhythmically; the motion of the hyoid bone is greater in swallowing than in processing cycles.

6.3.4 Swallowing Frequency

The cycle of swallowing is calculated to be 590 times in 24 hours: 146 cycles while eating, 394 cycles in between meals when awake, and 50 cycles while sleeping [46]. As the flow of saliva is less during sleep, there is less necessity for swallowing [47].

6.3.5 Teeth Contact During Swallowing

The mandible is balanced through teeth contact in the case of a typical adult swallow. Tooth gliding often happens in both chewing strokes: opening (55.9%) and closing (60.5%). The average glide length measured was 1 mm. There is a higher likelihood of the occurrence of gliding contacts if there is a higher lateral movement component during the closing stroke [22]. The mean tooth contact during the process of swallowing can last about 240–683 milliseconds, which is longer than thrice the duration of mastication [22, 48]. Also, the force that is put on the teeth during the process of swallowing is around 66.5 lbs, which is 7.8 lbs more than the force put on during the process of mastication [22]. It was found that the aggregate chewing and swallowing forces were approximately 100 N whereas the total maximal bite force in habitual occlusion amounted to 320 N [48]. Generally, 37% of the total maximal bite force is used while chewing and swallowing.

During swallowing, it is accepted that the mandible is supported and guided into the retruded position posteriorly [49]. An anterior glide takes place to the intercuspal position when the teeth do not fix cooperatively in this position. The closure of the mandible is maintained by reflex activities and muscle engrams. The masticatory muscles, during mastication, operate at a lesser activity level and in a much more harmonious manner when there is uniform teeth contact in the retruded closing position [50].

6.4 Speech

One of the vital functions of the masticatory system is speech. As the air is pushed from the lungs through the larynx and oral cavity by the diaphragm, speech comes out [2]. To reach the desired pitch of the sound, the laryngeal bands or vocal cords contract and relax in a controlled manner [51, 52]. When the pitch is produced, the resonance and exact sound articulation are determined by the precision assumed by the mouth. Since speech occurs when the air is released from the lungs, it is created during the expiration phase of the respiration [52]. Usually, inspiration is a fast process and happens either during a pause or end of a sentence. On the other hand, expiration is a prolonged process and allows the production of a series of words, phrases, or syllables.

Individuals can bring out different types of sounds with the use of lips and tongue to the palate and teeth [2, 51, 53, 54]. The union of these anatomic structures can also produce various sounds. The production of various sounds is shown in Figure 6.12 [2].

- Labiodental (Fricatives): These include "F", "V", and "Ph" sounds [55, 56]. They are produced between the maxillary incisors and the wet/dry line of the lower lips. They help to determine the position of incisal edges of maxillary teeth in complete denture fabrication.
- Linguoalveolar sounds (Sibilant): These include "S", "Z", "SH", "CH", and "J" [57, 58]. During the production of these sounds, the tip of the tongue contacts the anterior palate or the lingual surface of the teeth. While saying the "S" sound, there is a close approximation without touch between the maxillary and mandibular incisors with 1–1.5 mm interincisal separation. This is also known as the closest speaking speech. An "S" sound is created when the air is released from between the teeth.

K, G M B, P

F, V N T, D

S, CH NG, G TH, DH

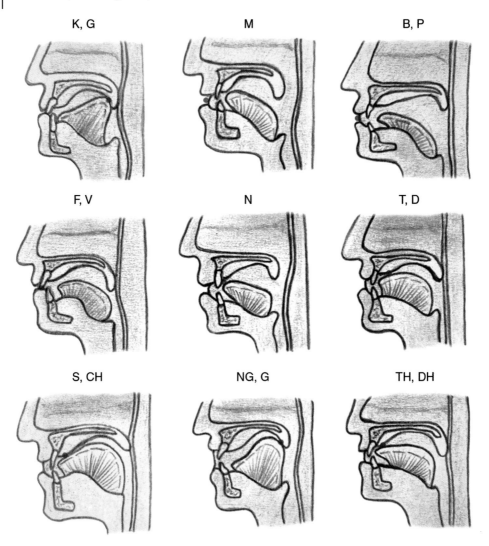

Figure 6.12 The specific positions of the teeth, lips, and tongue create articulation of sounds. Adapted from Reference [2]; chapter published in Management of Temporomandibular Disorders and Occlusion, 7th edition, Okeson J.P., Functional Neuroanatomy and Physiology of the Masticatory System, page 37, Copyright Elsevier (2013).

- Bilabial sounds: These sounds include "M", "B" and "P" sounds and are made by the lips. While making these sounds, the upper and lower lips contact each other [59, 60].
- Linguodental sounds: These sounds include "TH" and "T" [61]. To produce these sounds, the tip of the tongue comes into contact with the upper maxillary incisor or with contact upper and lower teeth.
- Guttural sounds: These sounds include "K" or "G" and these are produced when the posterior region of the tongue rises and touches the soft palate [2, 62].
- For producing the "D" sound, the tongue and the palate come into action. The tongue tip touches the palate behind the incisors [63].

Teaching correct articulation of sounds for speech starts from the initial stages of our life. Production of speech requires a combination of auditory, somatosensory, and motor information in the brain [64]. While the speech is occurring, teeth do not meet each other. But if there is tooth malposition and it contacts the opposing tooth while speaking, a message is immediately sent to the CNS through the sensory input of the tooth and periodontal ligament. The CNS retrieves this event as possible damage and quickly changes the pattern of the speech through the efferent nerve pathways. So, a new pattern of speech is made that avoids such contact with the tooth. The mandible is slightly deviated laterally because of this new speech pattern to bring out the required sound unaccompanied by tooth contact. When speech is learned, the process remains under the neuromuscular system's unconscious control or may be perceived as a learned reflex.

References

1 The glossary of prosthodontic terms: ninth edition. *J Prosthet Dent*, 2017. **117**: p. e1–e105.

2 Okeson, J.P., *Management of Temporomandibular Disorders and Occlusion*. 7th ed. 2013, St. Louis, Missouri: Mosby.

3 Nakata, M., Masticatory function and its effects on general health. *Int Dent J*, 1998. **48**(6): p. 540–548.

4 Kiliaridis, S., Masticatory muscle influence on craniofacial growth. *Acta Odontol Scand*, 1995. **53**(3): p. 196–202.

5 Enomoto, A., J. Watahiki, T. Yamaguchi, T. Irie, T. Tachikawa, and K. Maki, Effects of mastication on mandibular growth evaluated by microcomputed tomography. *Eur J Orthod*, 2010. **32**(1): p. 66–70.

6 Poikela, A., T. Kantomaa, M. Tuominen, and P. Pirttiniemi, Effect of unilateral masticatory function on craniofacial growth in the rabbit. *Eur J Oral Sci*, 1995. **103**(2): p. 106–111.

7 Kubo, K.Y., M. Iinuma, and H. Chen, Mastication as a stress-coping behavior. *Biomed Res Int*, 2015. **2015**: p. 876409.

8 Soeda, R., A. Tasaka, and K. Sakurai, Influence of chewing force on salivary stress markers as indicator of mental stress. *J Oral Rehabil*, 2012. **39**(4): p. 261–269.

9 Johnson, A.J., R. Jenks, C. Miles, M. Albert, and M. Cox, Chewing gum moderates multi-task induced shifts in stress, mood, and alertness. A re-examination. *Appetite*, 2011. **56**(2): p. 408–411.

10 Lund, J.P. and P.G. Dellow, The influence of interactive stimuli on rhythmical masticatory movements in rabbits. *Arch Oral Biol*, 1971. **16**(2): p. 215–223.

11 Lund, J.P., Mastication and its control by the brain stem. *Crit Rev Oral Biol Med*, 1991. **2**(1): p. 33–64.

12 Lundeen, H.C. and C.H. Gibbs, *Advances in Occlusion*. Vol. 14. 1982, Gainesville, Florida: John Wright Publisher.

13 Nishigawa, K., M. Nakano, E. Bando, and G.T. Clark, Effect of altered occlusal guidance on lateral border movement of the mandible. *J Prosthet Dent*, 1992. **68**(6): p. 965–969.

14 Gibbs, C.H., T. Messerman, J.B. Reswick, and H.J. Derda, Functional movements of the mandible. *J Prosthet Dent*, 1971. **26**(6): p. 604–620.

15 Pond, L.H., N. Barghi, and G.M. Barnwell, Occlusion and chewing side preference. *J Prosthet Dent*, 1986. **55**(4): p. 498–500.

16 Beyron, H., Occlusal relations and mastication in Australian aborigines. *Acta Odontol Scand*, 1964. **22**: p. 597–678.

17 Throckmorton, G.S., G.J. Groshan, and S.B. Boyd, Muscle activity patterns and control of temporomandibular joint loads. *J Prosthet Dent*, 1990. **63**(6): p. 685–695.

18 Christensen, L.V. and N.M. Rassouli, Experimental occlusal interferences. Part IV. Mandibular rotations induced by a pliable interference. *J Oral Rehabil*, 1995. **22**(11): p. 835–844.

19 Jankelson, B., G.M. Hoffman, and J.A. Hendron, Jr., The physiology of the stomatognathic system. *J Am Dent Assoc*, 1952. **46**(4): p. 375–386.

20 Adams, S.H., 2nd and H.A. Zander, Functional tooth contacts in lateral and in centric occlusion. *J Am Dent Assoc*, 1964. **69**: p. 465–473.

21 Glickman, I., J.H. Pameijer, F.W. Roeber, and M.A. Brion, Functional occlusion as revealed by miniaturized radio transmitters. *Dent Clin N Am*, 1969. **13**(3): p. 667–679.

22 Suit, S.R., C.H. Gibbs, and S.T. Benz, Study of gliding tooth contacts during mastication. *J Periodontol*, 1976. **47**(6): p. 331–334.

23 Mongini, F. and G. Tempia-Valenta, A graphic and statistical analysis of the chewing movements in function and dysfunction. *J Craniomandibular Pract*, 1984. **2**(2): p. 125–134.

24 Hernández-Vázquez, R.A., B. Romero-Ángeles, G. Urriolagoitia-Sosa, J.A. Vázquez-Feijoo, Á.J. Vázquez-López, and G. Urriolagoitia-Calderón, Numerical analysis of masticatory forces on a lower first molar considering the contact between dental tissues. *Appl Bionics Biomech*, 2018. **2018**: p. 4196343.

25 Bakke, M., Bite force and occlusion. *Semin Orthod*, 2006. **12**: p. 120–126.

26 Zhao, Y. and D. Ye, [Measurement of biting force of normal teeth at different ages]. *Hua Xi Yi Ke Da Xue Xue Bao*, 1994. **25**(4): p. 414–417.

27 Garner, L.D. and N.S. Kotwal, Correlation study of incisive biting forces with age, sex, and anterior occlusion. *J Dent Res*, 1973. **52**(4): p. 698–702.

28 Brekhus, P.J., W.D. Armstrong, and W.J. Simon, Stimulation of the muscles of mastication. *J Dent Res*, 1941. **20**(2): p. 87–92.

29 Gibbs, C.H., P.E. Mahan, A. Mauderli, H.C. Lundeen, and E.K. Walsh, Limits of human bite strength. *J Prosthet Dent*, 1986. **56**(2): p. 226–229.

30 Howell, A.H. and R.S. Manly, An electronic strain gauge for measuring oral forces. *J Dent Res*, 1948. **27**(6): p. 705–712.

31 Kiliaridis, S., M.G. Tzakis, and G.E. Carlsson, Effects of fatigue and chewing training on maximal bite force and endurance. *Am J Orthod Dentofacial Orthop*, 1995. **107**(4): p. 372–378.

32 Michael, C.G., N.S. Javid, F.A. Colaizzi, and C.H. Gibbs, Biting strength and chewing forces in complete denture wearers. *J Prosthet Dent*, 1990. **63**(5): p. 549–553.

33 Szyszka-Sommerfeld, L., A. Budzyńska, M. Lipski, S. Kulesza, and K. Woźniak, Assessment of masticatory muscle function in patients with bilateral complete cleft lip and palate and posterior crossbite by means of electromyography. *J Healthc Eng*, 2020. **2020**: p. 8828006.

34 Żmudzki, J., G. Chladek, and J. Kasperski, Biomechanical factors related to occlusal load transfer in removable complete dentures. *Biomech Model Mechanobiol*, 2015. **14**(4): p. 679–691.

35 Arksornnukit, M., T. Phunthikaphadr, and H. Takahashi, Pressure transmission and distribution under denture bases using denture teeth with different materials and cuspal angulations. *J Prosthet Dent*, 2011. **105**(2): p. 127–136.

36 Kijak, E., J. Margielewicz, D. Gąska, D. Lietz-Kijak, and W. Więckiewicz, Identification of mastication organ muscle forces in the biocybernetic perspective. *Biomed Res Int*, 2015. **2015**: p. 436595.

37 Matsuo, K. and J.B. Palmer, Anatomy and physiology of feeding and swallowing: normal and abnormal. *Phys Med Rehabil Clin N Am*, 2008. **19**(4): p. 691–707, vii.

38 Ruark, J.L., G.H. McCullough, R.L. Peters, and C.A. Moore, Bolus consistency and swallowing in children and adults. *Dysphagia*, 2002. **17**(1): p. 24–33.

39 Cleall, J.F., Deglutition: a study of form and function. *Am J Orthod*, 1965. **51**: p. 566–594.

40 Reynolds, E.W., F.L. Vice, and I.H. Gewolb, Variability of swallow-associated sounds in adults and infants. *Dysphagia*, 2009. **24**(1): p. 13–19.

41 Hiiemae, K.M. and J.B. Palmer, Food transport and bolus formation during complete feeding sequences on foods of different initial consistency. *Dysphagia*, 1999. **14**(1): p. 31–42.

42 Matsuo, K., K.M. Hiiemae, and J.B. Palmer, Cyclic motion of the soft palate in feeding. *J Dent Res*, 2005. **84**(1): p. 39–42.

43 Buettner, A., A. Beer, C. Hannig, and M. Settles, Observation of the swallowing process by application of videofluoroscopy and real-time magnetic resonance imaging-consequences for retronasal aroma stimulation. *Chem Senses*, 2001. **26**(9): p. 1211–1219.

44 Palmer, J.B. and K.M. Hiiemae, Eating and breathing: interactions between respiration and feeding on solid food. *Dysphagia*, 2003. **18**(3): p. 169–178.

45 Hodgson, M., R.S. Linforth, and A.J. Taylor, Simultaneous real-time measurements of mastication, swallowing, nasal airflow, and aroma release. *J Agric Food Chem*, 2003. **51**(17): p. 5052–5057.

46 Flanagan, J.B., The 24-hour pattern of swallowing in man. *J Dent Res*, 1963. **42**(abstr 165): p. 1072.

47 Schneyer, L.H., W. Pigman, L. Hanahan, and R.W. Gilmore, Rate of flow of human parotid, sublingual and submaxillary secretions during sleep. *J Dent Res*, 1956. **35**: p. 109–114.

48 Lundgren, D. and L. Laurell, Occlusal force pattern during chewing and biting in dentitions restored with fixed bridges of cross-arch extension. I. Bilateral end abutments. *J Oral Rehabil*, 1986. **13**(1): p. 57–71.

49 Graf, H. and H.A. Zander, Tooth contact patterns in mastication. *J Prosthet Dent*, 1963. **13**: p. 1055–1066.

50 Ramfjord, S.P., Dysfunctional temporomandibular joint and muscle pain. *J Prosthet Dent*, 1961. **11**: p. 353–362.

51 Zhang, Z., Mechanics of human voice production and control. *J Acoust Soc Am*, 2016. **140**(4): p. 2614–2614.

52 Hirano, M., J. Ohala, and W. Vennard, The function of laryngeal muscles in regulating fundamental frequency and intensity of phonation. *J Speech Hear Res*, 1969. **12**(3): p. 616–628.

53 Bulycheva, E.A., V.N. Trezubov, U.V. Alpateva, and D.S. Bulycheva, Sound production in totally edentulous patients before and after prosthetic treatment. *J Prosthodont*, 2018. **27**(6): p. 528–534.

54 Runte, C., M. Lawerino, D. Dirksen, F. Bollmann, A. Lamprecht-Dinnesen, and E. Seifert, The influence of maxillary central incisor position in complete dentures on /s/ sound production. *J Prosthet Dent*, 2001. **85**(5): p. 485–495.

55 Kong, Y.Y., A. Mullangi, and K. Kokkinakis, Classification of fricative consonants for speech enhancement in hearing devices. *PLoS One*, 2014. **9**(4): p. e95001.

56 Kehoe, M. and M. Philippart de Foy, The development of alveolar and alveopalatal fricatives in French-speaking monolingual and bilingual children. *J Speech Lang Hear Res*, 2023. **66**(2): p. 475–502.

57 Icht, M. and B.M. Ben-David, Sibilant production in Hebrew-speaking adults: apical versus laminal. *Clin Linguist Phon*, 2018. **32**(3): p. 193–212.

58 Hamlet, S.L., B.L. Cullison, and M.L. Stone, Physiological control of sibilant duration: insights afforded by speech compensation to dental prostheses. *J Acoust Soc Am*, 1979. **65**(5): p. 1276–1285.

59 Kasuya, H., S. Takeuchi, S. Sato, and K. Kido, Articulatory parameters for the perception of bilabials. *Phonetica*, 1982. **39**(2–3): p. 61–70.

60 Laukkanen, A.M., P. Lindholm, E. Vilkman, K. Haataja, and P. Alku, A physiological and acoustic study on voiced bilabial fricative/beta:/as a vocal exercise. *J Voice*, 1996. **10**(1): p. 67–77.

61 Zaki Mahross, H. and K. Baroudi, Spectrogram analysis of complete dentures with different thickness and palatal rugae materials on speech production. *Int J Dent*, 2015. **2015**: p. 606834.

62 Subramanian, H.H., M. Arun, P.A. Silburn, and G. Holstege, Motor organization of positive and negative emotional vocalization in the cat midbrain periaqueductal gray. *J Comp Neurol*, 2016. **524**(8): p. 1540–1557.

63 Flege, J.E., M.J. Munro, and L. Skelton, Production of the word-final English /t/-/d/ contrast by native speakers of English, Mandarin, and Spanish. *J Acoust Soc Am*, 1992. **92**(1): p. 128–143.

64 Guenther, F.H., Cortical interactions underlying the production of speech sounds. *J Commun Disord*, 2006. **39**(5): p. 350–365.

7

Nervous System Regulating the Masticatory System

7.1 Introduction

Movement of various head and neck musculature is achieved by the precise movement of the mandible for effective functioning of the masticatory system [1]. A neuromuscular system consisting of nerves and muscles controls the masticatory system.

7.2 Anatomy and Function of the Neuromuscular System

The neuromuscular system has two important parts (i.e. neurologic structures and muscles). The neuromuscular system is composed of a neural circuit including motor neurons, sensory neurons, and skeletal muscle fibers [2]. They are essential for the movements of the body parts and posture. The following sections explain neurological structures.

7.2.1 Neurologic Structures

7.2.1.1 The Neuron
Neuron is a fundamental structural component of the nervous system, and it has a protoplasmic body (nerve cell body) and protoplasmic extensions (axons and dendrites). Nerve cell bodies are present in the gray matter of the central nervous system (CNS) and those nerve cells which are found outside the CNS are called ganglia. Nerve fiber is anchored together by numerous neurons. These neurons can transfer impulses like chemical and electrical along with their axes to pass both inside and outside of the CNS. Neurons can be afferent or efferent depending on their function. An afferent (sensory) neuron sends the nerve impulse in the direction of the CNS, while an efferent (motor) neuron sends the impulse from the CNS to peripheral tissues. The initial sensory neuron is termed the first-order or primary neuron. Interneurons that lie within the CNS are second- and third-order sensory neurons [1]. From one neuron to another, nerve impulses are transmitted only at a synaptic junction or synapse. All afferent junctions are located within the CNS's gray matter.

Introduction to the Masticatory System and Dental Occlusion, First Edition. Dinesh Rokaya.
© 2025 John Wiley & Sons Ltd. Published 2025 by John Wiley & Sons Ltd.

7.2.1.2 Sensory Receptors

Nearly all bodily tissues contain sensory receptors, which are neurological structures that transmit information to the CNS through afferent neurons. Various sensory receptors are distributed all over the masticatory system [1]. Exteroceptors are types of sensory receptors that are in external tissues like the skin and oral mucosa and that provide information about the exterior tissues. They are specific exteroceptors describing heat, cold, and light touch, and nociceptors the pain and discomfort receptors. The proprioceptors, which are distributed in all the musculoskeletal structures, are the receptors for the position and mobility of the mandibular structures.

Information from the tissues is transferred into the CNS, brainstem, and cortex for interpretation and then appropriate action is taken. Impulses are sent back from the higher centers to the peripheral efferent organ via the spinal cord for the intended action. The sensory receptor sends a signal to the main afferent neuron, also known as a first-order neuron. This is then conveyed to a synapse in the spinal cord's dorsal horn by a secondary (second-order) neuron (Figure 7.1). All primary afferent neuron cell bodies are in the dorsal root ganglia (DRG). Eventually, the impulse is conducted by the second-order neuron to the higher centers via the spinal cord. There can also be different versions of interneurons such as (third-order and fourth-order) that contribute to the transmission of the impulse to the higher centers. Interneurons provide a connection between the main afferent neuron and the efferent (primary motor) neuron, which allows the reflex arc movement.

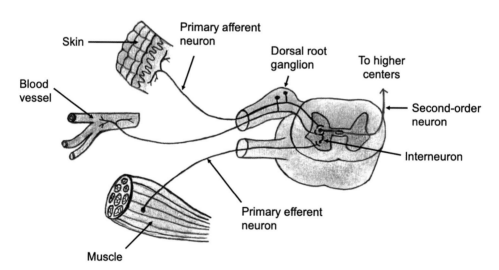

Figure 7.1 Impulse transfer. First-order (afferent) neurons convey information into the dorsal horn, where it synapses with second-order neurons, who then send it to higher centers. Adapted from Reference [1]; chapter published in Management of Temporomandibular Disorders and Occlusion, 7th edition, Okeson J.P., Functional Neuroanatomy and Physiology of the Masticatory System, page 22, Copyright Elsevier (2013).

7.2.1.3 Brainstem and Brain

Second-order neurons, once they receive the nerve impulse, transport them to higher-level centers for interpretation. Many interneurons may play a role in transmitting the impulses to higher centers [1, 3].

7.2.1.4 Spinal Tract Nucleus

Primary afferent neurons throughout the body establish synapses with second-order neurons in the spinal column's dorsal horn. The sensory impulse from the mouth and the face is transmitted by the trigeminal nerve and the fifth cranial nerve. Impulses relayed by the trigeminal nerve move to the areas of the pons where it communicates with the trigeminal spinal nucleus [1].

The brainstem trigeminal complex comprises (i) the primary sensory trigeminal nucleus (situated dorsally) that gets periodontal and some of the pulpal afferents, and (ii) the trigeminal nucleus spinal tract (located caudally). The spinal cord is categorized into three components: subnucleus oralis, subnucleus interpolaris, and subnucleus caudalis. Afferent nerves from the tooth pulp travel to all three subnuclei [4]. The subnucleus oralis is responsible for oral pain mechanisms [5–7] and the subnucleus caudalis is responsible for the nociceptive neurons [8, 9].

The motor nucleus of the fifth cranial nerve is another essential constituent of the trigeminal brainstem complex. This region is responsible for the interpretation of impulses for the motor responses [10, 11].

7.2.1.5 Reticular Formation

The interneurons send the signals up to the higher centers following the primary afferent neurons synapse in the spinal tract nucleus, with the help of a specific zone of the brainstem known as the reticular formation. They contain various concentrations of cells or nuclei "centers" that control the general activities of the brain either by stimulating or inhibiting the signals to the brain. They are also important for the pain and the sensory information.

7.2.1.6 Thalamus

The thalamus is situated in the middle of the brain, alongside the cerebrum and the midbrain. Nearly all signals from the lower parts of the brain and the spinal cord are communicated via thalamic synapses before they enter the cerebral cortex. The thalamus acts like a relay station for almost all the communication made among the brainstem, cerebellum, and cerebrum.

7.2.1.7 Hypothalamus

The hypothalamus represents a minor area situated in the center of the brain. It functions as an important center of the brain for maintaining body temperature, hunger, and thirst. It stimulates the sympathetic nervous system in the body, raising heart rate and causing blood artery constriction. A rise in psychological stress can excite the hypothalamus, causing it to stimulate the sympathetic nervous system and have a significant effect on nociceptive signals that reach the brain.

7.2.1.8 Limbic Structures

The limbic system comprises the cerebrum and diencephalon's border structures. They regulate bodily emotional and behavioral activities such as depression, anger, anxiety, and fear. They also act as a pain/pleasure center. In general, these impulses are not perceived consciously, but rather as a primitive instinct. Impulses transmitted from the limbic system to the hypothalamus can change the internal bodily mechanisms that are governed by the hypothalamus.

7.2.1.9 Cortex

The cerebral cortex, which is primarily composed of gray matter, represents the outermost region of the cerebrum. Despite being only 6 mm thick, the cerebral cortex includes 50–80 billion nerve cell bodies. These nerve impulses travel to different regions of the cortex, deeper brain areas, and the spinal cord. It is frequently linked to the thinking process and stores all our memories. Different regions of the cerebral cortex have different functions. The motor area controls our ability to attain many muscle skills. The sensory area receives somatosensory input. Within the cortex, there are the visual and auditory areas as well, which are special senses.

7.2.2 Muscles

7.2.2.1 Motor Unit

The motor unit represents the structural fundamental of a neuromuscular system (Figure 7.2) containing several muscle fibers innervated by one motor neuron. At a motor endplate, each neuron attaches to a muscle fiber. When a neuron fires, acetylcholine is released from the motor endplate, causing muscle fibers to depolarize. Depolarization will cause contraction of the muscle fibers.

One motor neuron innervates hundreds of muscle fibers. The more precise the movement, the fewer muscle fibers there are per motor neuron. In masticatory muscles, the number of muscle fibers per motor neuron differs. The inferior lateral pterygoid muscle has a moderately low ratio of muscle fibers to motor neurons and is excellent at fine regulations for horizontal mandibular position changes. The masseter, on the other hand, has a larger number of muscle fibers per motor neuron, which gives it the power for mastication.

Thousands of motor units are packed together with the help of connective tissue and fascia along with blood vessels and nerves to make up a muscle (Figure 7.3). The cervical spine and muscles support the skull and muscular forces maintain their desired position. There is a balance between the muscles that are connected to the anterior and posterior regions of the skull. Muscles that are attached to the posterior aspect skull consist of sternocleidomastoid, trapezius, splenius capitis, and longus capitis. To counteract these muscles, a group of muscles such as the masseter, the suprahyoids, and the infrahyoids are present in the anterior region of the head.

7.2.2.2 Muscle Function

The muscles in the human body function because of contraction and relaxation. When the motor units in the muscle are activated, muscle contraction is initiated. Isometric contractions occur when there is no change in the length of the muscle and there is no joint or limb

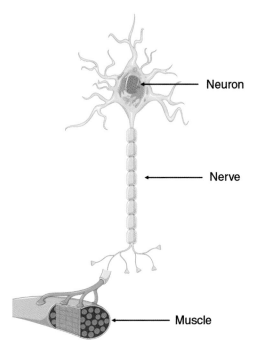

Figure 7.2 Neuromuscular junction. Adapted from Reference [12].

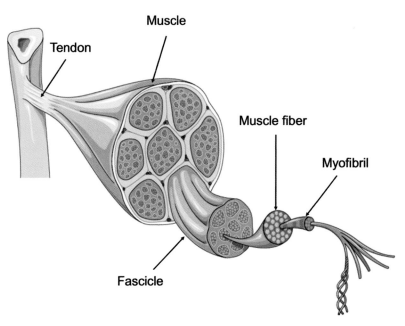

Figure 7.3 Muscle organization showing fascicle, muscle fiber, and myofibril. Adapted from Reference [12].

motion occurs. Whereas isotonic contractions occur when the muscle changes length, producing limb motion. Isotonic contraction occurs under a constant load. For example, the contraction of the masseter causes the mandible to raise up, pushing the teeth through a bolus of food. Specific motor units contract in response to a particular stimulus to maintain or stabilize the jaw. A muscle can also operate by regulated relaxation. When the stimulus is withdrawn, the motor unit's fibers relax and revert to their usual length.

During mastication, while the new food is put in the mouth, the masseter muscle relaxes in a controlled way. The muscles of the head and neck use these three functions to maintain a constant desirable head position. When the head is twisted to the right, some muscles must contract (isotonic contraction), others must undergo relaxation (controlled relaxation), and additional muscles must balance (isometric contraction).

7.2.2.3 Muscle Sensory Receptors
There are four primary sense sensors in the masticatory system, just like in the other musculoskeletal systems (proprioceptors): (i) Muscle spindles (primary sensory organs in the muscles). (ii) Golgi tendon organs (in the tendons). (iii) Pacinian corpuscles (in the tendons, joints, periosteum, fascia, and subcutaneous tissues). (iv) Nociceptors (in the tissues of the masticatory system).

7.2.2.4 Muscle Spindles
Skeletal muscles comprise two different forms of muscle fiber, namely extrafusal fiber and intrafusal fiber. Most of the muscle is made up of contractile extrafusal fiber, while intrafusal fiber contracts quite minutely. A muscle spindle is the name given to a cluster of intrafusal muscle fibers that are linked together by a connective tissue sheath (Figure 7.4).

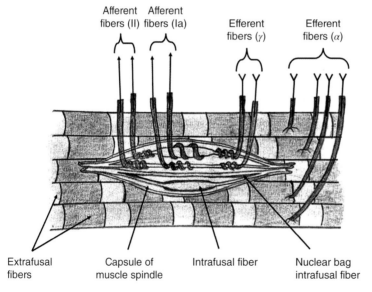

Figure 7.4 Muscle spindle. Adapted from Reference [1]; chapter published in Management of Temporomandibular Disorders and Occlusion, 7th edition, Okeson J.P., Functional Neuroanatomy and Physiology of the Masticatory System, page 22, Copyright Elsevier (2013).

They are arranged parallel with the extrafusal fibers and monitor the tension in the skeletal muscles. Each spindle's intrafusal fiber nuclei are organized in either a chainlike (nuclear-chain type) or grouped manner (nuclear-bag type).

Fusimotor nerve fibers provide efferent input to the intrafusal fibers. The CNS is the source of the efferent fibers and the gamma efferent fibers, and when these fibers are stimulated, they cause the intrafusal fibers to constrict. Their cell nuclei are mostly located in the trigeminal motor nucleus.

7.2.2.5 Golgi Tendon Organs

The Golgi tendon organelles are found between the muscle fibers and the bone in the muscular tendon. During normal function, they are more perceptive and active in the regulation of reflexes. They safeguard the muscle from damage or excessive strain. They are arranged in series with extrafusal muscle fibers. Each of these sensitive organs is made up of tendinous fibers that are encased in a fibrous cylinder and are surrounded by lymph cavities. Afferent fibers reach the organ close to the center and disperse throughout the fiber extension.

7.2.2.6 Pacinian Corpuscles

The pacinian corpuscles are big ovoid structures composed of connective tissue lamellae that are concentric. These are widely dispersed and contribute to the perception of motion and firm pressure. Various connective tissues including joints, tendons, periosteum, tendon insertions, fascia, and subcutaneous tissue contain these corpuscles.

7.2.2.7 Nociceptors

Nociceptors represent sensory receptors that are activated by an injury and send information about the injury (called "nociception") to the CNS via afferent nerve fibers. Nociceptors are found across the masticatory system's tissues. They react to a variety of general categories, including noxious mechanical and thermal stimuli, tactile responses to noxious injury, and low-threshold sensors for touch, pressure, or facial hair movement. Moreover, nociceptors (along with proprioceptors) are primarily responsible for monitoring the condition, location, and movement of masticatory system tissues.

7.3 Neuromuscular Function

7.3.1 Function of the Sensory Receptors

The capability of sensory receptors to provide feedback facilitates the dynamic equilibrium of the muscles of the head and neck region. The spindles transmit information to the CNS when a muscle is stretched gradually. Muscle contraction is controlled by the muscle spindles and Golgi tendon structures. Pacinian corpuscles are stimulated by the movement of the joints and tendons. All the sense organs always send the information to the CNS. The thalamus and brainstem monitor controlling and managing bodily functions. At this level, information about normal body homeostasis is allotted.

7.3.2 Reflex Action

A reflex action signifies a reaction to a stimulus transmitted as an impulse along an afferent neuron to a posterior nerve root or its cranial counterpart, then it is transported to an efferent neuron that travels back to the skeletal muscle [13, 14]. There is no cortical or brainstem impact on this reaction.

A reflex action can be either polysynaptic or monosynaptic. A monosynaptic response is also known as muscle stretch reflex or deep tendon reflex, and this happens when the afferent fiber in the CNS immediately activates the efferent fiber. The monosynaptic stretch reflex provides direct communication between sensory and motor neurons innervating the muscle [15]. A polysynaptic reflex takes place when there is stimulation of one or more interneurons in the CNS by afferent neurons. The polysynaptic stretch reflex synapses on interneurons within the spinal cord gray matter, which allows communication to multiple muscles for contraction or inhibition [15]. These two basic reflex responses, significant in the orofacial region, are the nociceptive reflex and myotatic reflex.

7.3.3 Nociceptive (Flexor) Reflex

The nociceptive reflex, also known as the flexor reflex, is a polysynaptic response that occurs in response to noxious stimulation, allowing for painful stimuli to activate an appropriate withdrawal response [16, 17]. This response is activated in the masticatory system when a hard item is abruptly experienced during mastication (Figure 7.5). The abruptly increased biting force applied to the molar immediately overloads the periodontal

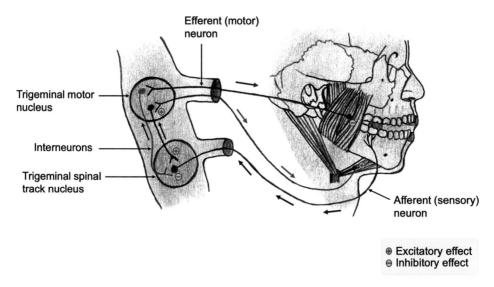

Figure 7.5 The nociceptive response is triggered by the abrupt biting of a hard object, and the noxious stimulation is triggered when the teeth and periodontal ligament are strained. Adapted from Reference [1]; chapter published in Management of Temporomandibular Disorders and Occlusion, 7th edition, Okeson J.P., Functional Neuroanatomy and Physiology of the Masticatory System, page 29, Copyright Elsevier (2013).

structures, resulting in a noxious sensation. This information is carried by primary afferent nerve impulses to the trigeminal spinal tract nucleus, where it synapses with interneurons. These interneurons move to the motor nucleus of the trigeminal nerve. Here, the movement of numerous groups of muscles must be synchronized for the intended motor response [18, 19]. Not only the elevator muscles must be inhibited but the muscles that open the jaw must be triggered to move the teeth away from possible injury [20, 21].

Two distinct actions take place as the afferent input from the sensory receptors hits the interneurons. Efferent neurons in the trigeminal motor nucleus of the jaw-opening muscles are activated via excitatory interneurons. This action leads to the contraction of these muscles. Simultaneously, the afferent fibers activate inhibitory interneurons, causing the jaw-raising muscles to relax. The consequence is that the jaw rapidly lowers, and the teeth are pulled away from the noxious stimulus-causing object (antagonistic inhibition).

7.3.4 Myotatic (Stretch) Reflex

The myotatic or stretch reflex is only a monosynaptic jaw response. This reflex refers to the contraction of a muscle in response to its passive stretching by increasing its contractility as long as the stretch is within physiological limits [22]. The stretching of a skeletal muscle produces a protective reflex by the contraction of the stretched muscle, for example, a patellar or knee-jerk reflex [23]. The myotatic reflex is also seen in the masticatory system. It can be observed in the masseter muscle when the chin is suddenly pressed downward with a tiny rubber hammer. Figure 7.6 shows the myotatic reflex and sequence of events. The myotatic reflex is established when a force is applied down on the chin. This causes the elevator muscles (masseter) to contract and the jaw to elevate into occlusion. The sequence of events goes as follows: the afferent output is increased, and impulses travel to the brainstem through the mesencephalic nucleus of the trigeminal nerve. In the trigeminal motor nucleus, the afferent fibers connect with the alpha efferent motor neurons, which then leads back to the elevator muscle's extrafusal fibers and these fibers constrict, which have been previously stretched.

In a clinical setting, relaxing the mouth muscles can demonstrate this reflex followed by slightly separating the teeth. A sharp downward touch on the chin reflexively lifts the jaw resulting in contraction of the masseter leading to tooth contact. As a result, the myotatic reflex occurs in the absence of a particular response from the brain.

7.3.5 Reciprocal Innervation

Controlling antagonistic muscles is critical in reflex movement. Each muscle that holds the head and partially regulates function, like other muscle systems, has an antagonist that inhibits its action. The mandible can be elevated and lowered by two distinct sets of muscles. Relaxing and lengthening the suprahyoid muscles permits the masseter, temporal, or medial pterygoid muscles to elevate the mandible. Similarly, the suprahyoid muscles must contract while the elevators relax and elongate for the mandible to be depressed. This neurologic regulating system for these antagonistic groups is termed reciprocal innervation. This process makes it possible to regulate mandibular movement precisely and smoothly. Additionally, each antagonistic

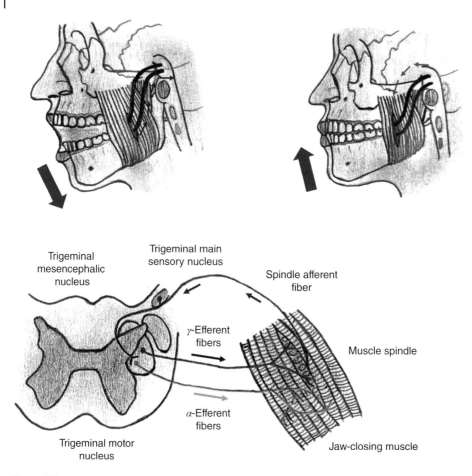

Figure 7.6 Myotatic reflex and sequence of events. Adapted from Reference [1]; chapter published in Management of Temporomandibular Disorders and Occlusion, 7th edition, Okeson J.P., Functional Neuroanatomy and Physiology of the Masticatory System, page 28, Copyright Elsevier (2013).

muscle group maintains a continuous posture of moderate tonus to maintain the skeletal connection of the neck, mandible, and skull.

7.4 Aging of the Neuromuscular System and Performance

Age-related changes occur in the neuromuscular system, including motor unit morphology and properties, which can lead to impaired motor performance. These can lead to (i) reduced muscle strength and increased fatigability, and (ii) increased variability during and between motor tasks and increased variability of contraction velocity and torque [2]. The major age-related changes in motor units at the level of the motor neuron, neuromuscular junction (NMJ), and muscle fiber [2].

Aging is also associated with a decrease in neurophysiological functions and age-related changes in the NMJ [24–26]. The NMJ plays an important role in musculoskeletal functions. Various factors such as oxidative stress, mitochondrial dysfunction, inflammation, changes in the innervation of muscle fibers, and properties of the motor units lead to the degeneration of NMJ and muscle mass and strength decline in aging [24, 26, 27]. Morphological and physiological changes result in a remodeling of the motor unit and a decline in the number of motor neurons (especially type II muscle fibers). These changes lead to the uncoupling of excitation–contraction and a decrease in communication between the muscular and nervous systems. Figure 7.7 shows the causes of dysfunction of NMJ with age and Figure 7.8 shows the age-related degenerative changes at NMJ [24].

A study by Hunter et al. [2] found that older women, who are generally weaker than similar-aged men, were vulnerable to increased fatigability and loss of steadiness during upper limb sustained contractions when cognitive demand was increased. Similarly, Pereira et al. [28] studied if higher cognitive demands (CD), stratified by sex, increased fatigability in older adults (>60 years). They found that the older women showed a significant increase in fatigability when low or high CD was imposed during sustained static contractions with the elbow flexor muscles. These all can affect the work-related motor tasks requiring high mental activity in aging.

It has been shown that the occlusal force is related to physical activities such as walking speed, balance function, muscle strength, and falls [29–34]. Yoshimoto et al. [35] did a study to determine the effect of walking training on oral health status by comparing the control group vs the intervention group. The intervention group underwent walking training (interval walking training) for at least five to six months. The walking training was done of five sets of fast walking above 70% peak aerobic capacity for walking for three minutes,

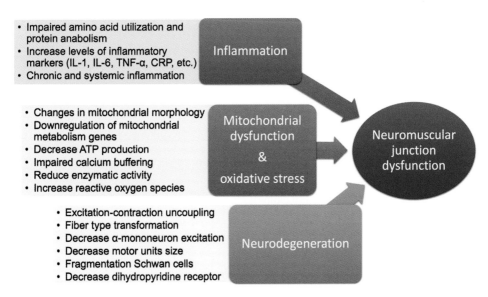

Figure 7.7 Causes of dysfunction of neuromuscular junction (NMJ) with age. IL = Interleukin, TNF = tumor necrosis factor, CRP = C-reactive protein, ATP = Adenosine triphosphate.

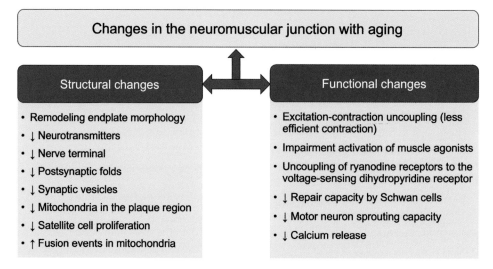

Figure 7.8 Age-related degenerative changes at neuromuscular junction (NMJ).

followed by three minutes of slow walking at ~40% peak aerobic capacity for walking per day for more than four days/week. The oral health status was evaluated for tongue pressure, masticatory performance, number of teeth, occlusal force, and salivary occult blood. It was found that walking training can help maintain and improve the occlusal force in both middle-aged and older people.

References

1 Okeson, J.P., *Management of Temporomandibular Disorders and Occlusion.* 7th ed. 2013, St. Louis, Missouri: Mosby.

2 Hunter, S.K., H.M. Pereira, and K.G. Keenan, The aging neuromuscular system and motor performance. *J Appl Physiol (1985)*, 2016. **121**(4): p. 982–995.

3 Guyton, A.C., *Textbook of Medical Physiology.* 8th ed. 1991, Philadelphia: Saunders.

4 De Laat, A., Reflexes elicitable in jaw muscles and their role during jaw function and dysfunction: a review of the literature. Part II. Central connections of orofacial afferent fibers. *Cranio*, 1987. **5**(3): p. 246–253.

5 Sessle, B.J., The neurobiology of facial and dental pain: present knowledge, future directions. *J Dent Res*, 1987. **66**(5): p. 962–981.

6 Sessle, B.J., Neural mechanisms and pathways in craniofacial pain. *Can J Neurol Sci*, 1999. **26**: p. S7–S11.

7 Sessle, B.J., Recent insights into brainstem mechanisms underlying craniofacial pain. *J Dent Educ*, 2002. **66**(1): p. 108–112.

8 Dubner, R. and G.J. Bennett, Spinal and trigeminal mechanisms of nociception. *Annu Rev Neurosci*, 1983. **6**: p. 381–418.

9 Iwata, K. and M. Shinoda, Role of neuron and non-neuronal cell communication in persistent orofacial pain. *J Dent Anesth Pain Med*, 2019. **19**(2): p. 77–82.

10 Lund, J.P., R. Donga, C.G. Widmer, and C.S. Stohler, The pain-adaptation model: a discussion of the relationship between chronic musculoskeletal pain and motor activity. *Can J Physiol Pharmacol*, 1991. **69**(5): p. 683–694.

11 Arendt-Nielsen, L. and T. Graven-Nielsen, Muscle pain: sensory implications and interaction with motor control. *Clin J Pain*, 2008. **24**(4): p. 291–298.

12 Neuromuscular junction. *Server Medical Art*. https://smart.servier.com/ (*Accessed on March 8, 2024*). 2023.

13 Fischer, D.B. and R.D. Truog, What is a reflex? A guide for understanding disorders of consciousness. *Neurology*, 2015. **85**(6): p. 543–548.

14 Brooks, C.M. and G. Lange, Patterns of reflex action, their autonomic components, and their behavioral significance. *Pavlov J Biol Sci*, 1982. **17**(2): p. 55–61.

15 Walkowski, A.D. and S. Munakomi, *Monosynaptic reflex*, in *StatPearls*. 2023, Treasure Island (FL): StatPearls Publishing.

16 Skljarevski, V. and N.M. Ramadan, The nociceptive flexion reflex in humans — review article. *Pain*, 2002. **96**(1–2): p. 3–8.

17 Linde, L.D., F.C. Duarte, H. Esmaeili, A. Hamad, K. Masani, and D.A. Kumbhare, The nociceptive flexion reflex: a scoping review and proposed standardized methodology for acquisition in those affected by chronic pain. *Br J Pain*, 2021. **15**(1): p. 102–113.

18 Tsai, C.M., C.Y. Chiang, X.M. Yu, and B.J. Sessle, Involvement of trigeminal subnucleus caudalis (medullary dorsal horn) in craniofacial nociceptive reflex activity. *Pain*, 1999. **81**(1–2): p. 115–128.

19 Tsai, C., The caudal subnucleus caudalis (medullary dorsal horn) acts as an interneuronal relay site in craniofacial nociceptive reflex activity. *Brain Res*, 1999. **826**(2): p. 293–297.

20 Stohler, C.S. and M.M. Ash, Excitatory response of jaw elevators associated with sudden discomfort during chewing. *J Oral Rehabil*, 1986. **13**(3): p. 225–233.

21 Hagberg, C., Electromyography and bite force studies of muscular function and dysfunction in masticatory muscles. *Swed Dent J Suppl*, 1986. **37**: p. 1–64.

22 Bhattacharyya, K.B., The stretch reflex and the contributions of C David Marsden. *Ann Indian Acad Neurol*, 2017. **20**(1): p. 1–4.

23 Eccles, R.M. and A. Lundberg, Integrative pattern of Ia synaptic actions on motoneurones of hip and knee muscles. *J Physiol*, 1958. **144**(2): p. 271–298.

24 Gonzalez-Freire, M., R. de Cabo, S.A. Studenski, and L. Ferrucci, The neuromuscular junction: aging at the crossroad between nerves and muscle. *Front Aging Neurosci*, 2014. **6**: p. 208.

25 Pratt, J., G. De Vito, M. Narici, and C. Boreham, Neuromuscular junction aging: a role for biomarkers and exercise. *J Gerontol A Biol Sci Med Sci*, 2021. **76**(4): p. 576–585.

26 Jang, Y.C. and H. Van Remmen, Age-associated alterations of the neuromuscular junction. *Exp Gerontol*, 2011. **46**(2–3): p. 193–198.

27 Li, Y., Y. Lee, and W.J. Thompson, Changes in aging mouse neuromuscular junctions are explained by degeneration and regeneration of muscle fiber segments at the synapse. *J Neurosci*, 2011. **31**(42): p. 14910–14919.

28 Pereira, H.M., V.C. Spears, B. Schlinder-Delap, T. Yoon, A. Harkins, K.A. Nielson, M. Hoeger Bement, and S.K. Hunter, Sex differences in arm muscle fatigability with cognitive demand in older adults. *Clin Orthop Relat Res*, 2015. **473**(8): p. 2568–2577.

29 Goto, T. and T. Ichikawa, Relationship between declines of physical performances and consciousness in elderly: occlusal force, grip strength, and walking speed. *J Jpn Acad Occulusion Health*, 2019. **25**: p. 39–43.

30 Kono, R., Relationship between occlusal force and preventive factors for disability among community-dwelling elderly persons. *Nihon Ronen Igakkai Zasshi*, 2009. **46**(1): p. 55–62.

31 Eto, M. and S. Miyauchi, Relationship between occlusal force and falls among community-dwelling elderly in Japan: a cross-sectional correlative study. *BMC Geriatr*, 2018. **18**(1): p. 111.

32 Lee, C.H.J., H. Vu, and H.D. Kim, Gender and age group modified association of dental health indicators with total occlusal force among Korean elders. *BMC Oral Health*, 2021. **21**(1): p. 571.

33 Kim, H.Y., M.S. Jang, C.P. Chung, D.I. Paik, Y.D. Park, L.L. Patton, and Y. Ku, Chewing function impacts oral health-related quality of life among institutionalized and community-dwelling Korean elders. *Community Dent Oral Epidemiol*, 2009. **37**(5): p. 468–476.

34 Yamashita, Y., N. Kogo, N. Kawaguchi, and N. Mizota, The relationship between the occlusal force and physical function in the frail elderly. *Jpn J Health Promot Phys Ther*, 2015. **5**: p. 129–133.

35 Yoshimoto, T., Y. Hasegawa, M. Furihata, A. Yoshihara, M. Shiramizu, M.T. Sta Maria, S. Hori, M. Morikawa, P. Marito, N. Kaneko, K. Nohno, H. Nose, S. Masuki, and T. Ono, Effects of interval walking training on oral health status in middle-aged and older adults: a case-control study. *Int J Environ Res Public Health*, 2022. **19**(21): p. 114465.

8

Bruxism and Clenching

8.1 Introduction

The movements of the jaw that are not associated with the function, or more precisely, not associated with facial expression, mastication, speech, swallowing, and postures of the jaw, with and without tooth contact, are described as parafunction. These include bruxism (grinding) and clenching. Such parafunctional habits, which can occur during the daytime and at night, have a great impact on the etiopathogenesis of temporomandibular disorders (TMD) [1]. However, the effect size and pattern of interaction with nocturnal activities are not yet clear.

8.2 Bruxism

Bruxism is a parafunctional grinding of teeth. According to Glossary of Prosthodontic Terms 9 (GPT-9), it may also be described as an oral habit that consists of involuntary rhythmic or spasmodic nonfunctional grinding, or clenching of teeth, other than chewing movements of the mandible, which may lead to occlusal trauma [2].

8.2.1 Types of Bruxism

According to the basis of occurrence, bruxism may be divided into awake bruxism or sleep bruxism (Figure 8.1) [3]. The prevalence of bruxism is reported by 20% in the adult population and during sleep, the awareness of tooth grinding is reported by 8% of the population [4]. Sleep bruxism is a behavior that was recently classified as a 'sleep-related movement disorder' [4].

8.2.2 Causes and Risk Factors

The cause behind this is usually believed to be numerous, although mostly undetermined. Some studies have shown important psychosocial risk factors for bruxism, mostly stress and anxiety, and this confirmation is rising [4–6]. Emotional or psychological stress has been regarded as a triggering point [7, 8]. Various studies found that awake and sleep

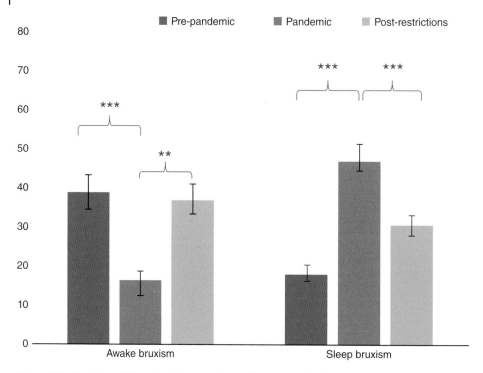

Figure 8.1 Awake and sleep bruxism prevalence for pre-pandemic, pandemic, and post-restriction groups. *** = $p < 0.001$, ** = $p < 0.01$. Adapted from Reference [3].

bruxism is associated with TMD [1, 9–11]. A study by Sierwald et al. [1] found that clenching or grinding while awake was seen in 33.9% of the TMD patients compared to only 11.2% in the controls (p < 0.001). Nocturnal clenching or grinding was seen in 49.4% of the TMD patients and 23.5% of the controls (p < 0.001). A study showed that females showed higher risks for bruxism only, but males showed higher risk with a combination of bruxism and TMD, and only TMD (Figure 8.2) [12].

A systematic review found that there is a positive association of bruxism with genetic factors, quality of life (school, emotional functions, and overuse of screen time), mother's anxiety and family conformation, diet, sleep behaviors, and sleep breathing disorders [13].

8.2.3 Pathophysiology

Awake bruxism is associated with nervous tic and is related to stress [4]. Although the pathology and physiology of awake bruxism are unknown, stress and anxiety are major risk factors.

Normally, the functional activity that happens in jaws is composed of properly monitored, rhythmic relaxation, and contraction of the muscles that allow sufficient flow of blood, which delivers oxygen to the tissues and removes the by-products collected at the cellular level. In contrast to this, bruxism develops a sustained muscle contraction for a

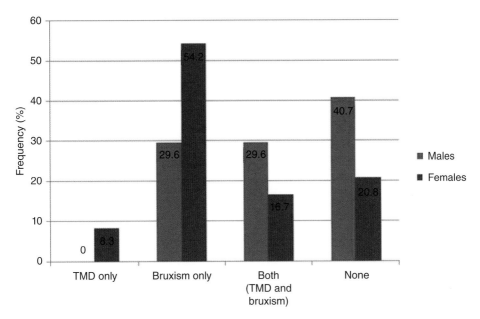

Figure 8.2 Bruxism, temporomandibular disorders (TMD), and bruxism with TMD in males and females. Reference [12] / MDPI / CC BY 4.0.

long duration of time [14]. In addition, this results in a decreased flow of blood, which further decreases the oxygen level in tissues of the muscle. Consequently, there is a rise of cellular by-products and carbon dioxide inside the tissues of muscle, which ultimately results in symptoms of pain, lethargy, and spasms [15, 16].

Bruxism involves the teeth, masticatory muscles, and nerve (trigeminal nerve), whose central nuclei include the mesencephalic trigeminal nucleus, which plays a significant role in the pathophysiology of bruxism [17]. The trigeminal nerve plays a significant role in bruxism, as it is involved in the pathophysiology of the disorder and can be stimulated by bruxism, leading to various effects on the body [18]. Conditions such as temporomandibular joint (TMJ) disorder, sleep bruxism, and orofacial dystonia may also affect the trigeminal nerve and contribute to the development of bruxism.

Moreover, the neuromuscular reflexes present in the event of functional activities protect the dental structures from injury. However, in the case of bruxism, this protective mechanism does not seem to be present, or the reflex threshold is somewhat increased, which results in a decreased impact on the activity of the muscle. Hence, the tooth contacts that usually impede the activity of muscle might not impede parafunctional activity. The measure of parafunctional activity is raised this way, which may result in the disruption of the associated structures [15].

Furthermore, bruxism is associated with alterations in the autonomic nervous system and stimulation of the trigeminal cardiac reflex (TCR) and can stimulate the TCR and lead to profound vagal effects on the heart. TCR is a well-established neurocardiogenic reflex that causes stimulation along the path of the fifth cranial nerve (trigeminal nerve) (Figure 8.3) [17].

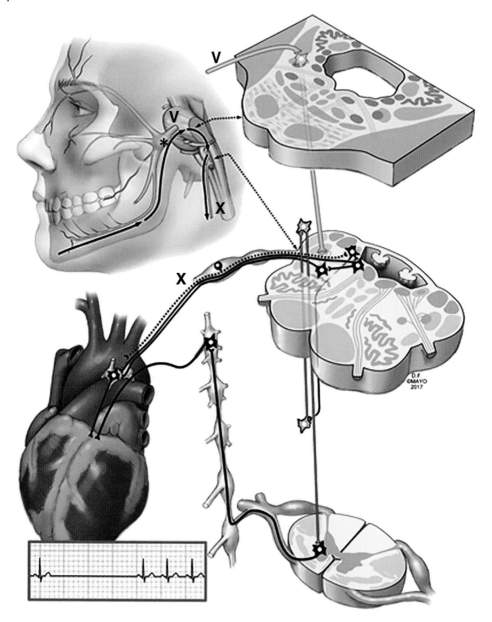

Figure 8.3 Trigeminal cardiac reflex. X = 5 motor nucleus of the vagus nerve, V = 5 trigeminal nerve, * = Gasserian ganglion. Reproduced from Reference [17] / with permission from Elsevier.

8.2.4 Clinical Features

Pain in the jaw and movement limitation are highly experienced by those patients who have sleep bruxism [14]. A frequent reason behind the wear of teeth due to attrition, mobile teeth, cusp fracture, alveolar exostoses, and muscular pain is bruxism [19]. Prolonged bruxism with clenching patients often shows severe linea alba of the cheek mucosae [20] as

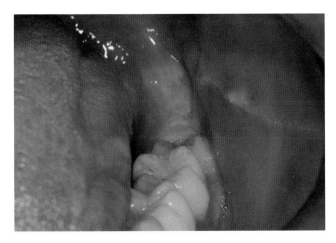

Figure 8.4 Clinical feature of prolonged bruxism with clenching showing severe linea alba of the cheek mucosae. Reference [20] / CC BY 4.0.

shown in Figure 8.4. Sleep bruxism and awake bruxism are often related to a malocclusion that advances toward TMJ pain and TMD [10, 11, 14]. Sleep bruxism is also associated with myofascial pain, arthralgia, and joint pathologies such as disc displacement and joint noises [21]. Khayat et al. [10] mentioned that deep overbite, and unilateral or bilateral posterior crossbite alone are not considered risk factors for bruxism or do not cause the pain associated with TMD and/or disc displacement.

8.2.5 Management

It is a challenge for the patient as well as the dentist to manage the disorders related to occlusion. The symptoms introduced by these conditions are often inconsistent, hence the diagnosis is arduous [22]. Hence, the therapy of bruxism is difficult and includes a multi-disciplinary approach [23]. Sleep bruxism can be properly diagnosed via patient report and clinical interview, clinical examination, or muscle activity [24]. Presently, no certain treatments have yet been identified that could terminate sleep bruxism. However, in the case of awake bruxism, specific behavior modification relaxation techniques, biofeedback massed therapy, habit awareness, and habit reversal therapy can put an end to it.

Several techniques have been suggested regarding the reduction of the detrimental effects of bruxism. Among them, the widely used technique is the application of various interocclusal appliances, i.e. occlusal splints, night guards, and mandibular advanced devices (MAD). It has been inferred that even though the interocclusal appliances are a convenient addition in managing sleep bruxism, they lack in providing curative/definitive treatment for bruxism or signs and symptoms of TMJ disorders [6, 16].

Figure 8.5 shows the management of a patient with bruxism with a splint made using 3D technology [25]. Digital technologies (intraoral scan and software) were used to fabricate a splint and 3D with clear resin. A 2.7 mm thick occlusal splint was fabricated, and the T-Scan system was used for the digital examination of the occlusion as shown in the Figure 8.6 [26]. The position of the TMJ components was proven radiologically.

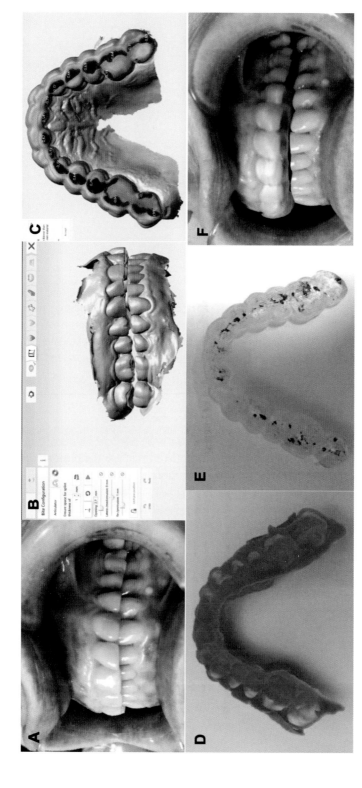

Figure 8.5 Fabrication of occlusal splint. A, Centric occlusion. B, Intermaxillary relation in software for the fabrication of the splint. C, Balanced occlusion from software. D, Silicone bite. E, Fabricated splint after occlusal adjustment. F, Splint in the patient's mouth. Reproduced from [25] / Shopova D et al. / CCBY 4.0.

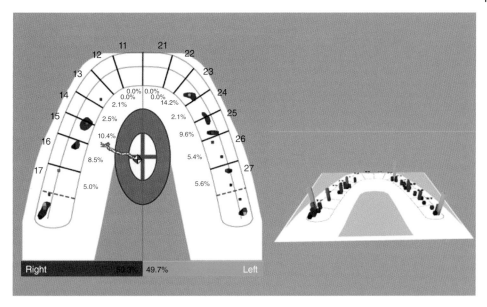

Figure 8.6 Occlusal registration in the T-scan software. Reference [26] / F1000 Research Ltd / CC BY 4.0.

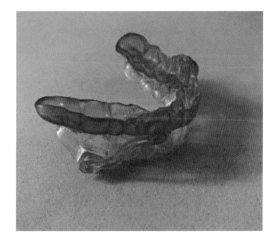

Figure 8.7 Single-unit mandibular protruding devices from Silensor-sl (Erkodent) showing the upper and lower dental arch splints with connectors. Reproduced from Reference [27] / with permission of Elsevier.

It showed that using digital technology allows for more accurate constructions and precise balancing of occlusal relationships.

The MAD can be of various types. Figure 8.7 shows Silensor-sl (Erkodent) single-unit mandibular protruding devices [27] and it consists of splints for the upper and lower dental arch splints with connectors in a registered constructive bite, which enables mouth breathing without obstruction. For this device, the bite is registered with the advanced mandibular position at 60% of the maximum protrusion. The splint covers the occlusal surfaces and incisal edges of all teeth extending to the alveolar mucosa.

Beddis et al. [24] mentioned that bruxism does not require treatment in itself, but the management is only indicated where problems arise from bruxism. They mentioned that oral appliances protect the teeth from damage caused by clenching/grinding, although they may reduce muscle activity. Behavioral strategies can be done and include biofeedback, relaxation, and improvement of sleep hygiene. Botox (botulinum toxin) administration to the masticatory muscles is found to reduce the frequency of bruxism but there are adverse effects. In another systematic review, they mentioned that the effective methods for management methods included oral appliance therapy with stabilization splints, cognitive-behavioral therapy, biofeedback therapy, and pharmacological therapy (clonazepam, rabeprazole, clonidine, and botox injection) [28]. The botulinum toxin type A is generally used in cosmetic medicine including for bruxism treatments. Intramuscular toxin injection causes proteolysis of synaptosomal-associated protein (SNAP-25), which is important for acetylcholine discharge at the neuromuscular junction [29]. This resets the action potential to zero and it causes the inhibition of muscle contraction resulting in paralysis of the muscle as shown in Figure 8.8 [29]. The effect of botulinum toxin gradually

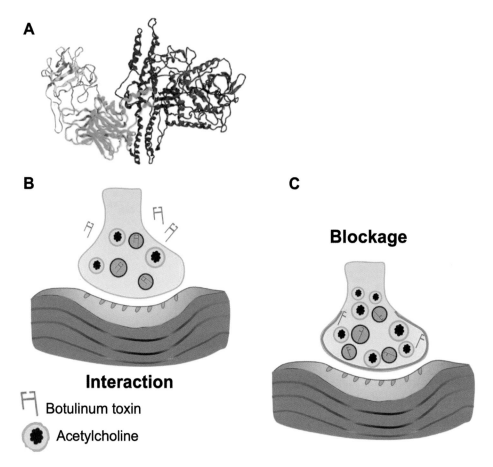

Figure 8.8 Botulinum toxin type A and its action in the inhibition of muscle contraction. A, Botulinum toxin. B, Binding of the toxin binds to presynaptic receptors and the active chain penetrates the cell through the disulfide bridges of the molecule. C, Once the botulinum toxin molecule is in the cytoplasm, the chains translocate inward to the cytosol and prevent the fusion of acetylcholine vesicles with the cytoplasmic membrane. Reference [29] / MDPI / CC BY 4.0.

degrades and disappears completely, generally after three months [29, 30]. In patients with a history of bruxism, masseter muscle hypertrophy occurs, the face looks puffy, and the mandibular jaw looks swollen because of the increased size of the muscle (Figure 8.9). Following the botulinum toxin injection, the masseter muscles can be normalized [29].

Finally, the optimal treatment strategies depend on a correct diagnosis that includes both the patient stress profile and precise analysis of the occlusion concerning the state and position of the TMJs [31, 32]. In addition, dentists should be aware of the etiology, pathophysiology, and latest advancements in the management strategies of bruxism.

8.3 Clenching

According to GPT-9, clenching can be defined as a pressing and clamping of the jaws and teeth together, frequently associated with acute nervous tension or physical effort [2].

8.3.1 Clinical Features

Teeth clenching may be a typical presentation of increased muscle tones associated with emotional stress. It may also happen while lifting heavy objects or during other activities that require physical pressure. Unusual clenching that occurs when there is no emotional or physical trigger is a type of bruxism (centric bruxism). Habitual clenching usually does not involve noticeable jaw movement, but teeth with deflective premature contacts may be moved or loosened by repeated clenching activity. Patients are rarely aware of their clenching habits [19].

Habitual clenching in the presence of deflective tooth interferences often leads to the typical symptoms of occluso-muscle pain [33]. Electromyography (EMG) evidence shows a decreased muscle activity level as well as a decreased proclivity to clench when all the deflective occlusal interferences are eliminated [34]. It is also a common occurrence for hypermobile teeth to tighten, following a precisely completed occlusal correction, even if the patient continues to clench [19]. Although the influence of the central nervous system in habitual clenching cannot be easily eliminated, it is always suggested for occlusal correction.

The occlusal interferences are also considered an etiologic factor in bruxing [19]. Occlusal interferences are a potent trigger for bruxing in patients under stress, but they are also potent triggers for many patients who do not have excessive stress in their lives. It is certainly true that the elimination of occlusal interference can normalize even the greater muscle activity levels that result from the most trivial-looking premature occlusal contacts [19].

It seems clear that occlusal triggers are a primary factor in eccentric bruxing. It is also clear that to damage the teeth, they must be in the way of border movements of the mandible. A perfected occlusion with posterior disocclusion makes it impossible to achieve excursive contact on posterior teeth if the anterior guidance is stable. There is no tendency to brux on anterior teeth unless they interfere with the patient's envelope of function. The exception to this is certain types of dystonia from CNS-related etiologies. Although, in most cases, eccentric bruxing can be diminished or terminated, a successful termination of clenching is not yet predictable.

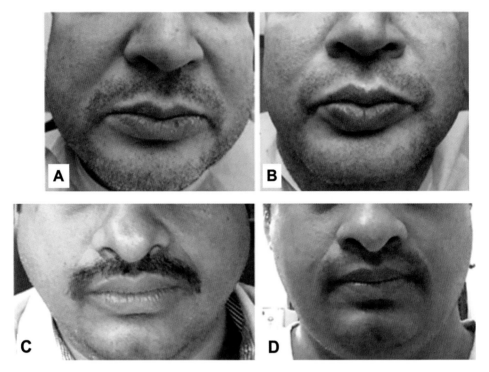

Figure 8.9 Botox injections in the masseter muscle. A and C, Patient before the injection. B and D, Patient after the injection at 40 days. Reproduced from Reference [29] / Zhang et al / CC BY 4.0.

References

1 Sierwald, I., M.T. John, O. Schierz, C. Hirsch, D. Sagheri, P.G. Jost-Brinkmann, and D.R. Reissmann, Association of temporomandibular disorder pain with awake and sleep bruxism in adults. *J Orofac Orthop*, 2015. **76**(4): p. 305–317.

2 Ferro, K.J. The glossary of prosthodontic terms: ninth edition. *J Prosthet Dent*. 2017. **117**: p. e1–e105.

3 Osses-Anguita Á.E., T. Sánchez-Sánchez, X.A. Soto-Goñi, M. García-González, F. A. Fariñas, R. Cid-Verdejo, E.A. Sánchez Romero, and L. Jiménez-Ortega, Awake and sleep bruxism prevalence and their associated psychological factors in first-year university students: a pre-mid-post COVID-19 pandemic comparison. *Int J Environ Res Public Health*, 2023. **20**(3): p. 2452.

4 Lavigne, G.J., S. Khoury, S. Abe, T. Yamaguchi, and K. Raphael, Bruxism physiology and pathology: an overview for clinicians. *J Oral Rehabil*, 2008. **35**(7): p. 476–494.

5 Manfredini, D. and F. Lobbezoo, Role of psychosocial factors in the etiology of bruxism. *J Orofac Pain*, 2009. **23**(2): p. 153–166.

6 Shetty, S., V. Pitti, C.L. Satish Babu, G.P. Surendra Kumar, and B.C. Deepthi, Bruxism: a literature review. *J Indian Prosthodont Soc*, 2010. **10**(3): p. 141–148.

7 Sampaio, N.M., M.C. Oliveira, A.C. Andrade, L.B. Santos, M. Sampaio, and A. Ortega, Relationship between stress and sleep bruxism in children and their mothers: a case control study. *Sleep Sci*, 2018. **11**(4): p. 239–244.

8   Smardz, J., H. Martynowicz, A. Wojakowska, M. Michalek-Zrabkowska, G. Mazur, and M. Wieckiewicz, Correlation between sleep bruxism, stress, and depression-a polysomnographic study. *J Clin Med*, 2019. **8**(9): p. 1344.

9   Huhtela, O.S., R. Näpänkangas, T. Joensuu, A. Raustia, K. Kunttu, and K. Sipilä, Self-reported bruxism and symptoms of temporomandibular disorders in Finnish University students. *J Oral Facial Pain Headache*, 2016. **30**(4): p. 311–317.

10 Khayat, N., E. Winocur, A. Emodi Perelman, P. Friedman-Rubin, Y. Gafni, and N. Shpack, The prevalence of posterior crossbite, deep bite, and sleep or awake bruxism in temporomandibular disorder (TMD) patients compared to a non-TMD population: a retrospective study. *Cranio*, 2021. **39**(5): p. 398–404.

11 Raphael, K.G., M.N. Janal, D.A. Sirois, B. Dubrovsky, J.J. Klausner, A.C. Krieger, and G.J. Lavigne, Validity of self-reported sleep bruxism among myofascial temporomandibular disorder patients and controls. *J Oral Rehabil*, 2015. **42**(10): p. 751–758.

12 Peleg, O., L. Haddad, S. Kleinman, T. Sella Tunis, G. Wasserman, E. Mijiritsky, and Y. Oron, Temporomandibular disorders and bruxism in patients attending a tinnitus clinic. *Appl Sci*, 2022. **12**(10): p. 4970.

13 Restrepo-Serna, C. and E. Winocur, Sleep bruxism in children, from evidence to the clinic a systematic review. *Front Oral Health*, 2023. **4**: p. 1166091.

14 Reddy, S.V., M.P. Kumar, D. Sravanthi, A.H.B. Mohsin, and V. Anuhya, Bruxism: a literature review. *J Int Oral Health*, 2014. **6**(6): p. 105–109.

15 Okeson, J.P., *Management of Temporomandibular Disorders and Occlusion*. 7th ed. 2013, St. Louis, Missouri: Mosby.

16 Murali, R.V., P. Rangarajan, and A. Mounissamy, Bruxism: conceptual discussion and review. *J Pharm Bioallied Sci*, 2015. **7**(Suppl 1): p. S265–S270.

17 Sugrue, A., C.V. DeSimone, P. Gaba, M.A. El-Harasis, A.J. Deshmukh, and S.J. Asviravtham. Bruxism Stimulating the Trigeminal Cardiac Reflex. *HeartRhythm Case Rep*, 2018. **4**(8): 329–331.

18 Demjaha, G., B. Kapusevska, and B. Pejkovska-Shahpaska, Bruxism unconscious oral habit in everyday life. *Open Access Maced J Med Sci*, 2019. **7**(5): p. 876–881.

19 Dawson, P.E., *Functional Occlusion: From Tmj to Smile Design*. 2006, Edinburgh: Elsevier Mosby.

20 Bracci, A., F. Lobbezoo, B. Häggman-Henrikson, A. Colonna, L. Nykänen, M. Pollis, J. Ahlberg, D. Manfredini, I.N.f.O. Pain, and R.D. Methodology, Current knowledge and future perspectives on awake bruxism assessment: expert consensus recommendations. *J Clin Med*, 2022. **11**(17): p. 5083.

21 Jiménez-Silva, A., C. Peña-Durán, J. Tobar-Reyes, and R. Frugone-Zambra, Sleep and awake bruxism in adults and its relationship with temporomandibular disorders: a systematic review from 2003 to 2014. *Acta Odontol Scand*, 2017. **75**(1): p. 36–58.

22 Safari, A., Z. Jowkar, and M. Farzin, Evaluation of the relationship between bruxism and premature occlusal contacts. *J Contemp Dent Pract*, 2013. **14**(4): p. 616–621.

23 Kevilj, R., K. Mehulic, and A. Dundjer, Temporomandibular disorders and bruxism Part I. *Minerva Stomatol*, 2007. **56**(7–8): p. 393–397.

24 Beddis, H., M. Pemberton, and S. Davies, Sleep bruxism: an overview for clinicians. *Br Dent J*, 2018. **225**(6): p. 497–501.

25 Shopova, D., T. Bozhkova, S. Yordanova, and M. Yordanova, Case report: digital analysis of occlusion with T-scan novus in occlusal splint treatment for a patient with bruxism. *F1000Res*, 2021. **10**: 915.

26 Shopova, D., T. Bozhkova, S. Yordanova, and M. Yordanova, Case report: digital analysis of occlusion with T-Scan Novus in occlusal splint treatment for a patient with bruxism. *F1000Res*, 2021. **10**: 915.

27 Wojda, M. and J. Kostrzewa-Janicka, Influence of MAD application on episodes of obstructive apnea and bruxism during Sleep-A prospective study. *J Clin Med*, 2022. **11**(19): p. 5809.

28 Minakuchi, H., M. Fujisawa, Y. Abe, T. Iida, K. Oki, K. Okura, N. Tanabe, and A. Nishiyama, Managements of sleep bruxism in adult: a systematic review. *Jpn Dent Sci Rev*, 2022. **58**: p. 124–136.

29 Malcangi, G., A. Patano, C. Pezzolla, L. Riccaldo, A. Mancini, C. Di Pede, A.D. Inchingolo, F. Inchingolo, I.R. Bordea, G. Dipalma, and A.M. Inchingolo, Bruxism and botulinum injection: challenges and insights. *J Clin Med*, 2023. **12**(14): p. 4586.

30 Küçüker, İ., I.A. Aksakal, A.V. Polat, M.S. Engin, E. Yosma, and A. Demir, The effect of chemodenervation by botulinum neurotoxin on the degradation of hyaluronic acid fillers: an experimental study. *Plast Reconstr Surg*, 2016. **137**(1): p. 109–113.

31 Levitt, S.R., Predictive value of the TMJ scale in detecting clinically significant symptoms of temporomandibular disorders. *J Craniomandib Disord*, 1990. **4**(3): p. 177–185.

32 Dawson, P.E., A classification system for occlusions that relates maximal intercuspation to the position and condition of the temporomandibular joints. *J Prosthet Dent*, 1996. **75**(1): p. 60–66.

33 Granger, E.R., Occlusion in temporomandibular joint pain. *J Am Dent Assoc*, 1958. **56**: p. 659.

34 Adhikari, H., A. Kapoor, U. Prakash, and A. Srivastava, "Electromyographic pattern of masticatory muscles in altered dentition Part II". *J Conserv Dent*, 2011. **14**(2): p. 120–127.

9

Aging-Related Changes of Masticatory System

9.1 Introduction

Aging is a continuous process, and it causes susceptibility to diseases. World Health Organization (WHO) has denoted old age to be 60–65 years of age [1]. Forman et al. [2] divided old age into three age groups as follows:

- Young old: 60–69 years
- Middle old: 70–79 years
- Very old: 80 years and above

In the human body, age-related deterioration in the function of various organ systems, including the masticatory system, is shown in Figure 9.1 [3]. There is an underlying association of old age with mastication [4]. Various changes in the body and masticatory system occur with age which are explained in the following sections.

The masticatory function can be expressed in terms of masticatory performance and mastication ability [5]. Figure 9.2 shows the relationship between the various factors of the masticatory function, which includes the masseter muscle thickness, dental factors, bite force and occluding area, and age [6–9]. The dental factor is the main factor that influences masticatory function. The number of teeth and functional tooth units influences the bite force and occluding area, and these correlate with the masticatory performance [10]. It was found that keeping 20 or more natural teeth and at least eight functional tooth units is important in reducing the likelihood of self-assessed chewing difficulties [8]. Age has less direct influence on masticatory performance [11]. The posterior occlusal support is important in oral rehabilitation for masticatory function in the elderly [5].

Finally, the characteristics of food influence the masticatory functions [7, 12]. During mastication, food size is reduced, and saliva moistens the food and binds the food into a bolus that can be swallowed. Time is required to break the food and add the saliva to form a cohesive bolus. The jaw muscle activity helps in breaking solid food. Muscle response is important to maintain a constant chewing rhythm under varying food resistance conditions [7]. Dry and hard products require more chewing cycles before swallowing than moist and soft foods. In older adults, muscle function training and prosthetic treatments help to increase masticatory performance to improve overall health [13].

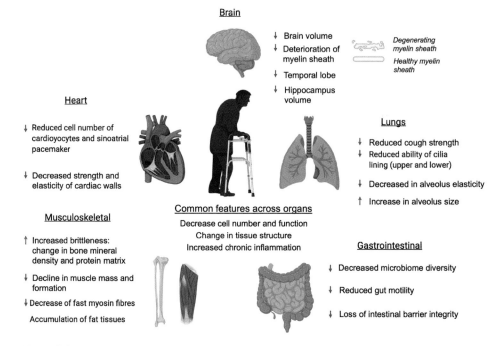

Figure 9.1 Age-related deterioration in function of various organ systems during human aging. Reference [3] / Springer Nature / CC BY 4.0.

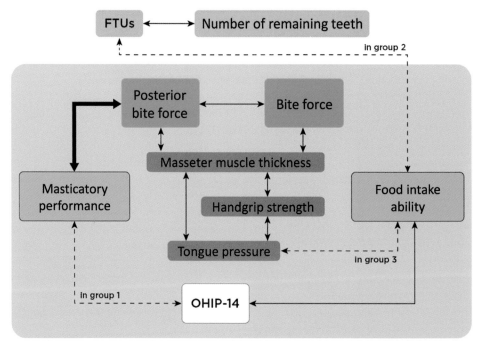

Figure 9.2 Relationship of the various factors of the masticatory function. Reference [5] / MDPI / CC BY 4.0. FTU = functional tooth units.

9.2   Effect of Aging on Mastication

With age, the masticatory muscles mostly weaken, the elasticity of the swallowing mechanism may diminish, and loss of dentition decreases the bite force and masticatory performance [14]. Also, the cross-section areas of masticatory muscles, especially masseters and medial pterygoids, weaken in old age [15–17]. In addition, a reduction in both salivation and orosensory receptors, i.e. gustative and mechanical receptors, increases the sensory thresholds that affect reflex responsiveness and perception of food texture [14, 18, 19]. In complete denture patients, there was a reduction in the masticatory efficiency by 50–85% than the individuals with intact dentition [20]. In old age, due to a decrease in motor skills of the tongue and lack of muscle tones which have a role in masticatory movements also decreases the efficiency of mastication [21, 22].

Some adaptive changes occur with age and can still make a food bolus prepared for swallowing during healthy aging [14]. With healthy aging, an increased cycle of mastication is seen with maximal pulverization of food before swallowing [23]. An increase in three cycles per sequence every 10 years. A study found that despite the reduction in the muscle mass and maximal bite force, there was no difference in the electromyography (EMG) of temporalis muscles and masseter in aged individuals with full dentition chewing brittle foods [23]. The reason might be the enhancement of muscle fibers in comparison to the overall motor unit number. The masticatory rate is also found to remain constant throughout normal aging [23]. Aged individuals with acceptable oral well-being try to preserve their capability to make a food bolus for safe swallowing [24].

9.2.1   Dentation

With age, teeth loss occurs due to dental caries and periodontal disease. A negative effect of periodontal disease is seen with bite force and mastication efficiency. In addition, teeth wear might be important for masticatory efficiency due to an increase in the surface area of occlusal contact [14]. The contact between maxillary and mandibular teeth may improve in healthy dental arcades in the aging population as teeth wear occurs with time [25]. In elderly people, larger functional areas due to occlusal teeth wear help to preserve masticatory efficiency [26]. Singh et al. [27] mentioned that the number of teeth, loose teeth, and pain in the mouth were associated with chewing disability. In addition, fewer teeth and pain in the mouth contribute most to chewing function.

In another study, Käyser et al. [9] mentioned that there are two patterns of oral function changes: (i) oral functions that change slowly until four occlusal units are left and then change rapidly, and (ii) oral functions that change gradually without a sudden change. There is sufficient adaptive capacity to maintain adequate oral function in shortened dental arches when at least four occlusal units are left.

In a study, it was found that a coarser bolus is produced by denture wearers when compared to dentate subjects [28]. Despite their deficiency, denture wearers increase the masticatory cycles and total muscular activity to acclimatize their mastication to hard foods [29, 30]. But there is still impaired mastication to chew hard foods like raw carrots. Elderly denture wearers tend to replace teeth with implants or implant-retained dentures. These types of prostheses greatly improved mastication [31]. Masticatory performance and bite forces are also similar to the dentate control [32]. With aging, various oral functions are affected such as masticatory function, swallowing, oral occlusal force, mucosal wetness, and lip motor function including tongue motor function and tongue pressure (Figure 9.3) [33].

9.2.2 Salivation

The most common problem among aged individuals is dryness of the mouth. It has also been reported that the loss of a tooth induces xerostomia [32]. Taking medicines and therapies in an aging population may cause xerostomia, such as chemotherapy, radiotherapy,

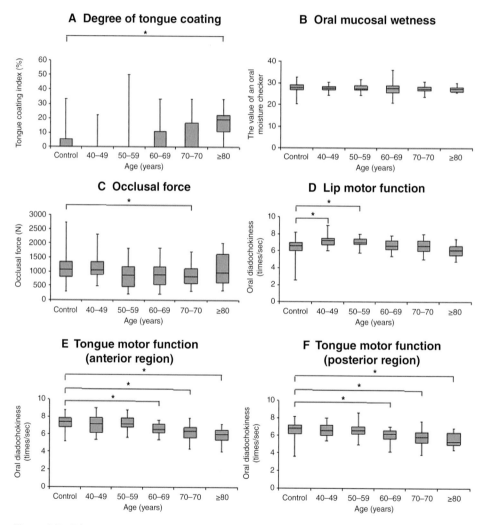

Figure 9.3 Decrease in various oral functions with aging. A, Degree of tongue coating. B, Oral mucosal wetness. C, Occlusal force. D, Lip motor function. E, Tongue motor function (anterior region). F, Tongue motor function (posterior region). G, Tongue pressure. H, Masticatory function. I, Swallowing function. Reference [33] / MDPI / CC BY 4.0.

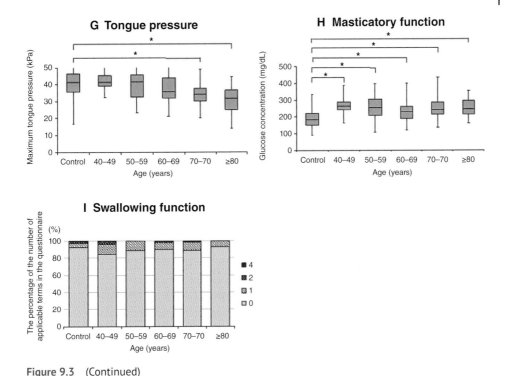

Figure 9.3 (Continued)

and psychotropic. Elderly persons may also suffer from autoimmune diseases like Sjögren's syndrome, where there is reduced saliva flow [34]. Xerostomia and other salivary supply dysfunctions may affect the masticatory process negatively making it difficult to make the bolus. In normal conditions, chewing increases the salivary flow rate as it is an adaptation of the masticatory activity [35]. Elderly adults reimburse their loss of teeth and/or muscular force by a longer chewing sequence, which increases the salivary flow and maintains its saliva output level till their life expectancy [36].

9.3 Effect of Aging on Masticatory Muscles

With age, there is a slow decrease in the volume and mass of the skeletal muscles mainly because of a decrease in the motor units, muscle fibers, and type two fibers [37]. In old age, progressive reduction in muscle strength and impaired mobility occurs, which affects mastication [32, 38]. Hence, exercise and strength training are beneficial to inverse the harmful outcome of weakness that is age-related.

Newton et al. [36], by using computed tomography, investigated the effects of old age and dental state on jaw muscles (the masseter and medial pterygoid). It showed a decrease in the area of both muscles with age when seen cross-sectionally, and females showed a lower distribution. In addition, with an increase in age, a substantial decrease in the compactness of the muscles was observed. This is accompanied by a reduction in the masticatory forces.

9.4   Effect of Aging on Swallowing

Aging causes a decrease in tactile sensations and a substantial reduction in perceptions of bolus viscosity due to a decrease in the number of sensory receptors or higher sensory thresholds of the sensory receptors that are related to age [32, 39].

Due to the aging process, all three stages of deglutition (oral, pharyngeal, and esophageal) are affected but often temporal modifications of these stages remain hardly noticeable in healthy individuals. Aging decreases muscle mass, which is associated with sarcopenia, which might be the reason for the reduction in the swallowing process [40]. Alterations in the cerebral white matter tracts are suggestive of a slowed swallowing syndrome or presbyphagia, which was detected using magnetic resonance imaging [41]. The pharyngeal stage of deglutition is slowed down and shortened when the pharyngoesophageal sphincter is opened, shortly thereby reducing peristalsis movements (amplitude and speed), weakened cough reflex, and hypotony of the vocal cords. Reduction in muscle strength is an influencing factor [40]. The esophagus stage of swallowing is less affected by aging. A few changes were seen at the superior esophageal sphincter, and they are: it takes longer time to relax after swallowing and there was some amendment in contraction pressure [42].

9.5   Effect of Aging on Temporomandibular Joint

The articular region of the mandibular condyle is enclosed within the cartilage which is mostly made of collagen fibers and proteoglycans. Hence, the viscoelastic response of temporomandibular joint (TMJ) permits the cartilage to act as a stress absorber throughout the function [43]. Condylar remodeling, which is a normal physiologic process, occurs in the structure of the TMJ that eventually adapts the TMJ to meet the functional stress [44]. Morphologically, severe degenerative changes are seen in the mandibular condyle, especially in the articular surface with increasing age [45]. An irregular surface on the cortical bone plate was most frequently seen at 50–60 years of age, and a flattened surface was mostly seen after 70 years of age in the radiographic investigation [45]. On histological examination, it is advocated that a reduction in the cellular components with increasing age might have an important role in the progress of degenerative changes.

The mandibular condylar cartilage (MCC), a fibrocartilaginous tissue comprising both type I and type II collagen, and the MCC, supports and distributes functional loads [46]. With advancing age, the serious change in the TMJ is that cartilage is replaced by bone [43]. The development of calcified cartilage is because of modification in the cellular composition, which may cause degenerative disorders of the TMJ. Osteoarthritis in aged individuals is believed to be caused by the disproportion between the factors that damage and the factors that prevent damage or repair the cartilage damage [43]. Osteoarthritis affects TMJ along with numerous other joints.

9.6   Effect of Aging on the Muscles and Nerves

With age, quantitative as well as qualitative changes in motor units occur. It has shown damage to alpha motor neurons of the spinal cord following their axon degeneration with increasing age [47, 48].

The EMG of muscles showed there were changes in the amplitude and duration of action potentials of motor units [49]. In addition, macro-EMG of the motor unit size showed a rise in the size of the motor unit (muscle fibers per motor unit) in numerous extremity muscles among individuals aged more than 60 years [50, 51]. It also showed that in aged individuals there was a decrease in motor unit numbers [52]. With age, there is a lessening in the number of motor units but a rise in the size of motor units [37]. Furthermore, with age, the fibers undergo denervation cycles followed by reinnervation, resulting from motor neuron death in the spinal cord or injury to axons of the peripheral nerve.

With aging, there is a decline in various oral functions [33, 53–55]. Senile muscle atrophy, also known as sarcopenia, is an age-related muscle atrophy due to a decrease in skeletal muscle mass with age-related decline in physical activities [56–59]. Considering this, musculo-skeletal improvement functions play an important intervention in preventing and improving sarcopenia and extending healthy life expectancy [60]. The relationship between physical function and occlusal force has been studied and has shown that occlusal force is related to physical activities such as walking speed, balance function, muscle strength, and falls [61–66].

Yoshimoto et al. [53] did a study to determine the effect of walking training on oral health status by comparing the control group vs the intervention group. The intervention group underwent walking training (interval walking training) for at least five to six months. The walking training was done of five sets of fast walking above 70% peak aerobic capacity for walking for three minutes, followed by three minutes of slow walking at ~40% peak aerobic capacity for walking per day for more than four days/week. The oral health status was evaluated for tongue pressure, masticatory performance, number of teeth, occlusal force, and salivary occult blood. It was found that walking training can help maintain and improve the occlusal force in both middle-aged and older people (Figure 9.4).

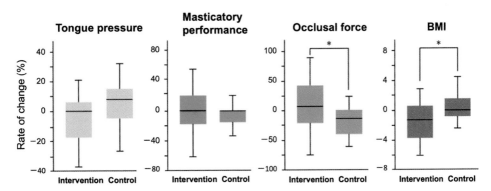

Figure 9.4 Tongue pressure, masticatory performance, occlusal force, and BMI in the interventional group (walking training) and control in middle-aged people. BMI = Body mass index. Reference [53] / MDPI / CC BY 4.0.

References

1 *WHO. United Nations. Definition of an older or elderly person.* http://wwwwhoint/ healthinfo/survey/ageingdefnolder/en/ *(Accessed on April 29, 2021).* 2014.

2 Forman, D.E., A.D. Berman, C.H. McCabe, D.S. Baim, and J.Y. Wei, PTCA in the elderly: the "young-old" versus the "old-old". *J Am Geriatr Soc*, 1992. **40**(1): p. 19–22.

3 Xu, W., G. Wong, Y.Y. Hwang, and A. Larbi, The untwining of immunosenescence and aging. *Semin Immunopathol*, 2020. **42**(5): p. 559–572.

4 Osterberg, T., G.E. Carlsson, K. Tsuga, V. Sundh, and B. Steen, Associations between self-assessed masticatory ability and some general health factors in a Swedish population. *Gerodontology*, 1996. **13**(2): p. 110–117.

5 Kim, S., R.M. Doh, L. Yoo, S.A. Jeong, and B.Y. Jung, Assessment of age-related changes on masticatory function in a population with normal dentition. *Int J Environ Res Public Health*, 2021. **18**(13): 6899.

6 Boretti, G., M. Bickel, and A.H. Geering, A review of masticatory ability and efficiency. *J Prosthet Dent*, 1995. **74**(4): p. 400–403.

7 van der Bilt, A., Assessment of mastication with implications for oral rehabilitation: a review. *J Oral Rehabil*, 2011. **38**(10): p. 754–780.

8 Ueno, M., T. Yanagisawa, K. Shinada, S. Ohara, and Y. Kawaguchi, Masticatory ability and functional tooth units in Japanese adults. *J Oral Rehabil*, 2008. **35**(5): p. 337–344.

9 Käyser, A.F., Shortened dental arches and oral function. *J Oral Rehabil*, 1981. **8**(5): p. 457–462.

10 Ikebe, K., K. Morii, K. Matsuda, and T. Nokubi, Discrepancy between satisfaction with mastication, food acceptability, and masticatory performance in older adults. *Int J Prosthodont*, 2007. **20**(2): p. 161–167.

11 Ikebe, K., K. Matsuda, R. Kagawa, K. Enoki, M. Yoshida, Y. Maeda, and T. Nokubi, Association of masticatory performance with age, gender, number of teeth, occlusal force and salivary flow in Japanese older adults: is ageing a risk factor for masticatory dysfunction? *Arch Oral Biol*, 2011. **56**(10): p. 991–996.

12 Pereira, L.J., M.B. Duarte Gaviao, and A. Van Der Bilt, Influence of oral characteristics and food products on masticatory function. *Acta Odontol Scand*, 2006. **64**(4): p. 193–201.

13 Kim, H.E., Influential factors of masticatory performance in older adults: a cross-sectional study. *Int J Environ Res Public Health*, 2021. **18**(8): p. 4286.

14 Mioche, L., P. Bourdiol, and M.A. Peyron, Influence of age on mastication: effects on eating behaviour. *Nutr Res Rev*, 2004. **17**(1): p. 43–54.

15 Newton, J.P., E.W. Abel, E.M. Robertson, and R. Yemm, Changes in human masseter and medial pterygoid muscles with age: a study by computed tomography. *Gerodontics*, 1987. **3**(4): p. 151–154.

16 Bakke, M., B. Holm, B.L. Jensen, L. Michler, and E. Möller, Unilateral, isometric bite force in 8-68-year-old women and men related to occlusal factors. *Scand J Dent Res*, 1990. **98**(2): p. 149–158.

17 Hatch, J.P., R.S. Shinkai, S. Sakai, J.D. Rugh, and E.D. Paunovich, Determinants of masticatory performance in dentate adults. *Arch Oral Biol*, 2001. **46**(7): p. 641–648.

18 Navazesh, M., R.A. Mulligan, V. Kipnis, P.A. Denny, and P.C. Denny, Comparison of whole saliva flow rates and mucin concentrations in healthy Caucasian young and aged adults. *J Dent Res*, 1992. **71**(6): p. 1275–1278.

19 Smith, A., C.M. Weber, J. Newton, and M. Denny, Developmental and age-related changes in reflexes of the human jaw-closing system. *Electroencephalogr Clin Neurophysiol*, 1991. **81**(2): p. 118–128.

20 Liedberg, B., K. Stoltze, and B. Owall, The masticatory handicap of wearing removable dentures in elderly men. *Gerodontology*, 2005. **22**: p. 10–16.

21 Carlsson, G.E., Bite force and chewing efficiency. *Front Oral Physiol*, 1974. **1**(0): p. 265–292.

22 Koshino, H., T. Hirai, T. Ishijima, and Y. Ikeda, Tongue motor skills and masticatory performance in adult dentates, elderly dentates, and complete denture wearers. *J Prosthet Dent*, 1997. **77**(2): p. 147–152.

23 Peyron, M.A., O. Blanc, J.P. Lund, and A. Woda, Influence of age on adaptability of human mastication. *J Neurophysiol*, 2004. **92**(2): p. 773–779.

24 Feldman, R.S., K.K. Kapur, J.E. Alman, and H.H. Chauncey, Aging and mastication: changes in performance and in the swallowing threshold with natural dentition. *J Am Geriatr Soc*, 1980. **28**(3): p. 97–103.

25 Lee, S.-M., S. Oh, S.J. Yu, K.-M. Lee, S.-A. Son, Y.H. Kwon, and Y.-I. Kim, Association between brain lateralization and mixing ability of chewing side. *J Dent Sci*, 2017. **12**(2): p. 133–138.

26 Bourdiol, P., S. Abou El Karam, J.F. Martin, E. Nicolas, and L. Mioche, Age and gender-related differences in premolar and molar functional areas. *J Oral Rehabil*, 2007. **34**(4): p. 251–258.

27 Singh, K.A. and D.S. Brennan, Chewing disability in older adults attributable to tooth loss and other oral conditions. *Gerodontology*, 2012. **29**(2): p. 106–110.

28 Slagter, A.P., L.W. Olthoff, F. Bosman, and W.H. Steen, Masticatory ability, denture quality, and oral conditions in edentulous subjects. *J Prosthet Dent*, 1992. **68**(2): p. 299–307.

29 Veyrune, J.L., C. Lassauzay, E. Nicolas, M.A. Peyron, and A. Woda, Mastication of model products in complete denture wearers. *Arch Oral Biol*, 2007. **52**(12): p. 1180–1185.

30 Wayler, A.H., M.E. Muench, K.K. Kapur, and H.H. Chauncey, Masticatory performance and food acceptability in persons with removable partial dentures, full dentures and intact natural dentition. *J Gerontol*, 1984. **39**(3): p. 284–289.

31 Feine, J.S. and J.P. Lund, Measuring chewing ability in randomized controlled trials with edentulous populations wearing implant prostheses. *J Oral Rehabil*, 2006. **33**(4): p. 301–308.

32 Peyron, M.A., A. Woda, P. Bourdiol, and M. Hennequin, Age-related changes in mastication. *J Oral Rehabil*, 2017. **44**(4): p. 299–312.

33 Iyota, K., S. Mizutani, S. Oku, M. Asao, T. Futatsuki, R. Inoue, Y. Imai, and H. Kashiwazaki, A cross-sectional study of age-related changes in oral function in healthy Japanese individuals. *Int J Environ Res Public Health*, 2020. **17**(4): 1376.

34 Nagler, R.M. and O. Hershkovich, Sialochemical and gustatory analysis in patients with oral sensory complaints. *J Pain*, 2004. **5**(1): p. 56–63.

35 Bourdiol, P., L. Mioche, and S. Monier, Effect of age on salivary flow obtained under feeding and non-feeding conditions. *J Oral Rehabil*, 2004. **31**(5): p. 445–452.

36 Newton, J.P., R. Yemm, R.W. Abel, and S. Menhinick, Changes in human jaw muscles with age and dental state. *Gerodontology*, 1993. **10**(1): p. 16–22.

37 Porter, M.M., A.A. Vandervoort, and J. Lexell, Aging of human muscle: structure, function and adaptability. *Scand J Med Sci Sports*, 1995. **5**(3): p. 129–142.

38 Kieser, J., G. Jones, G. Borlase, and E. MacFadyen, Dental treatment of patients with neurodegenerative disease. *N Z Dent J*, 1999. **95**(422): p. 130–134.

39 Logemann, J.A., Effects of aging on the swallowing mechanism. *Otolaryngol Clin N Am*, 1990. **23**(6): p. 1045–1056.

40 Shaker, R. and I.M. Lang, Effect of aging on the deglutitive oral, pharyngeal, and esophageal motor function. *Dysphagia*, 1994. **9**(4): p. 221–228.

41 Robbins, J., J.W. Hamilton, G.L. Lof, and G.B. Kempster, Oropharyngeal swallowing in normal adults of different ages. *Gastroenterology*, 1992. **103**(3): p. 823–829.

42 Dejaeger, E., W. Pelemans, E. Ponette, and E. Joosten, Mechanisms involved in postdeglutition retention in the elderly. *Dysphagia*, 1997. **12**(2): p. 63–67.

43 Kuroda, S., K. Tanimoto, T. Izawa, S. Fujihara, J.H. Koolstra, and E. Tanaka, Biomechanical and biochemical characteristics of the mandibular condylar cartilage. *Osteoarthr Cartil*, 2009. **17**(11): p. 1408–1415.

44 Mathew, A.L., A.A. Sholapurkar, and K.M. Pai, Condylar changes and its association with age, TMD, and dentition status: a cross-sectional study. *Int J Dent*, 2011. **2011**: p. 413639.

45 Ishibashi, H., Y. Takenoshita, K. Ishibashi, and M. Oka, Age-related changes in the human mandibular condyle: a morphologic, radiologic, and histologic study. *J Oral Maxillofac Surg*, 1995. **53**(9): p. 1016–1023.

46 Orajärvi, M., S. Laaksonen, R. Hauru, E. Mursu, E. Jonaviciute, H.M. Voipio, A. Raustia, and P. Pirttiniemi, Changes in type I and type II collagen expression in rat mandibular condylar cartilage associated with aging and dietary loading. *J Oral Facial Pain Headache*, 2018. **32**(3): p. 258–265.

47 Maxwell, N., R.W. Castro, N.M. Sutherland, K.L. Vaughan, M.D. Szarowicz, R. de Cabo, J.A. Mattison, and G. Valdez, α-Motor neurons are spared from aging while their synaptic inputs degenerate in monkeys and mice. *Aging Cell*, 2018. **17**(2): p. e12726.

48 Hepple, R.T. and C.L. Rice, Innervation and neuromuscular control in ageing skeletal muscle. *J Physiol*, 2016. **594**(8): p. 1965–1978.

49 Howard, J.E., K.C. McGill, and L.J. Dorfman, Age effects on properties of motor unit action potentials: ADEMG analysis. *Ann Neurol*, 1988. **24**(2): p. 207–213.

50 Piasecki, M., A. Ireland, D.A. Jones, and J.S. McPhee, Age-dependent motor unit remodelling in human limb muscles. *Biogerontology*, 2016. **17**(3): p. 485–496.

51 Henderson, R.D. and P.A. McCombe, Assessment of motor units in neuromuscular disease. *Neurotherapeutics*, 2017. **14**(1): p. 69–77.

52 Watanabe, K., A. Holobar, M. Kouzaki, M. Ogawa, H. Akima, and T. Moritani, Age-related changes in motor unit firing pattern of vastus lateralis muscle during low-moderate contraction. *Age*, 2016. **38**(3): p. 48.

53 Yoshimoto, T., Y. Hasegawa, M. Furihata, A. Yoshihara, M. Shiramizu, M.T. Sta Maria, S. Hori, M. Morikawa, P. Marito, N. Kaneko, K. Nohno, H. Nose, S. Masuki, and T. Ono, Effects of interval walking training on oral health status in middle-aged and older adults: a case-control study. *Int J Environ Res Public Health*, 2022. **19**(21): 14465.

54 Watanabe, Y., H. Hirano, H. Arai, S. Morishita, Y. Ohara, A. Edahiro, M. Murakami, H. Shimada, T. Kikutani, and T. Suzuki, Relationship between frailty and oral function in community-dwelling elderly adults. *J Am Geriatr Soc*, 2017. **65**(1): p. 66–76.

55 Okamoto, N., K. Tomioka, K. Saeki, J. Iwamoto, M. Morikawa, A. Harano, and N. Kurumatani, Relationship between swallowing problems and tooth loss in community-dwelling independent elderly adults: the Fujiwara-kyo study. *J Am Geriatr Soc*, 2012. **60**(5): p. 849–853.

56 Evans, W.J. and W.W. Campbell, Sarcopenia and age-related changes in body composition and functional capacity. *J Nutr*, 1993. **123**(2 Suppl): p. 465–468.

57 Vu, H., P.T. Vo, and H.D. Kim, Gender modified association of oral health indicators with oral health-related quality of life among Korean elders. *BMC Oral Health*, 2022. **22**(1): p. 168.

58 Walston, J.D., Sarcopenia in older adults. *Curr Opin Rheumatol*, 2012. **24**(6): p. 623–627.

59 Larsson, L., H. Degens, M. Li, L. Salviati, Y.I. Lee, W. Thompson, J.L. Kirkland, and M. Sandri, Sarcopenia: aging-related loss of muscle mass and function. *Physiol Rev*, 2019. **99**(1): p. 427–511.

60 Beckwée, D., A. Delaere, S. Aelbrecht, V. Baert, C. Beaudart, O. Bruyere, M. de Saint-Hubert, and I. Bautmans, Exercise interventions for the prevention and treatment of Sarcopenia. A systematic umbrella review. *J Nutr Health Aging*, 2019. **23**(6): p. 494–502.

61 Goto, T. and T. Ichikawa, Relationship between declines of physical performances and consciousness in elderly: occlusal force, grip strength, and walking speed. *J Jpn Acad Occulusion Health*, 2019. **25**: p. 39–43.

62 Kono, R., Relationship between occlusal force and preventive factors for disability among community-dwelling elderly persons. *Nihon Ronen Igakkai Zasshi*, 2009. **46**(1): p. 55–62.

63 Eto, M. and S. Miyauchi, Relationship between occlusal force and falls among community-dwelling elderly in Japan: a cross-sectional correlative study. *BMC Geriatr*, 2018. **18**(1): p. 111.

64 Lee, C.H.J., H. Vu, and H.D. Kim, Gender and age group modified association of dental health indicators with total occlusal force among Korean elders. *BMC Oral Health*, 2021. **21**(1): p. 571.

65 Kim, H.Y., M.S. Jang, C.P. Chung, D.I. Paik, Y.D. Park, L.L. Patton, and Y. Ku, Chewing function impacts oral health-related quality of life among institutionalized and community-dwelling Korean elders. *Community Dent Oral Epidemiol*, 2009. **37**(5): p. 468–476.

66 Yamashita, Y., N. Kogo, N. Kawaguchi, and N. Mizota, The relationship between the occlusal force and physical function in the frail elderly. *Jpn J Health Promot Phys Ther*, 2015. **5**: p. 129–133.

10

Occlusal Concept and Its Application in Various Fields

10.1 Introduction

In dental practice, patients may present with painful teeth, loose teeth, excessive wear, orofacial pain, and temporomandibular joint (TMJ) disorders. Achieving predictable functional treatment is dependent on a good occlusion [1]. Good occlusal harmony results in the following things [1]:

- Accurate treatment planning
- Restoration longevity
- Patient comfort
- Improved esthetics

Therefore, occlusal therapy can be accomplished through restorative dental procedures to treat temporomandibular joint disorder (TMD), because these procedures alter occlusion.

Generally, restorative dental procedures fall into two categories: operative dentistry and fixed prosthodontics. Most restorations in operative dentistry are made up intraorally (for example, an amalgam or a composite resin). Whereas in fixed prosthodontics, most of the restorations are fabricated extraoral and cementation is done in the mouth (for example, inlay, onlay, full crown, and fixed partial denture) [2].

10.2 Articulators

The articulator simulates the patient's mandibular movements and provides static and dynamic relationships to observe malocclusions or dysfunctionalities extra orally [3, 4]. According to the Glossary of Prosthodontic Terms 9 (GPT-9), an articulator is a mechanical instrument that represents the TMJs and jaws, to which maxillary and mandibular casts may be attached to simulate some or all mandibular movements of teeth [5]. There are four types of articulators as follows [5, 6].

- Class I articulator (nonadjustable articulator) – A simple instrument that is capable of single static registration and vertical motion. For example, simple hinge articulator (Figure 10.1).

Introduction to the Masticatory System and Dental Occlusion, First Edition. Dinesh Rokaya.
© 2025 John Wiley & Sons Ltd. Published 2025 by John Wiley & Sons Ltd.

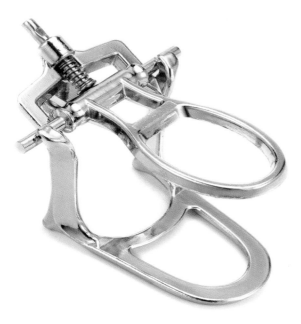

Figure 10.1 Simple hinge nonadjustible articulator.

- Class II articulator – An instrument that permits horizontal as well as vertical motion but does not orient the motion to the TMJs.
- Class III articulator (semiadjustible articulator) – An instrument that simulates condylar pathways by using averages or mechanical equivalents for all or part of the motion. These instruments allow for the orientation of the casts relative to the joints and may be arcon or nonarcon instruments which are discussed below. For example, Hanau™ Wide-Vue arcon articulator and Balance 105 nonarcon articulator from Hager Werken (Figure 10.2).
- Class IV articulator (fully adjustable) – An instrument that will accept 3D dynamic registrations; these instruments allow for orientation of the casts to the TMJs and simulation of mandibular movements. For example, the Dinar® D5A articulator (Figure 10.3).

Arcon articular has a glenoid cavity located in the upper branch and a condyle in the lower branch [5]. Their condylar articulation movement is equal to human articulation. They are the most recommended for beginners. For example, Hanau™ Wide-Vue arcon articulator (Figure 10.2A).

Nonacron has condyles in the upper part of the articulator and the glenoid cavity in the lower part of the instrument [5]. For example, Balance 105 articulator from Hager Werken (Figure 10.2B).

At present, virtual articulators are being used in computer software [7, 8]. The virtual articulator generates the animated movements of the mandible based on the input data through the code [9]. They substitute mechanical articulators and avoid their errors and help dentists, dental technicians, and dental prosthetists to provide individualized

A

B

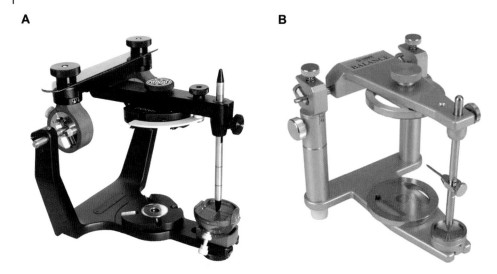

Figure 10.2   Arcon and nonarcon type of semiadjustible articulators. A, Hanau™ Wide-vue arcon articulator. B, Balance 105 nonarcon articulator from Hager Werken.

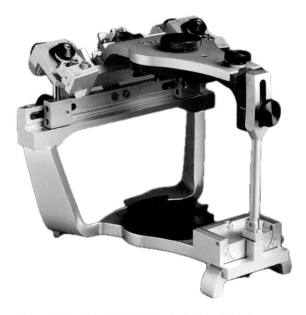

Figure 10.3   Dinar® D5A fully adjustable articulator.

treatment for each patient [10]. In addition, they have the advantage of performing the full analysis in static and dynamic occlusion through dynamic visualization in 3D of the mandible, the maxilla, or both in various body planes [9]. In addition, virtual articulators are used for the analysis of complex static and dynamic occlusal relations. They require 3D

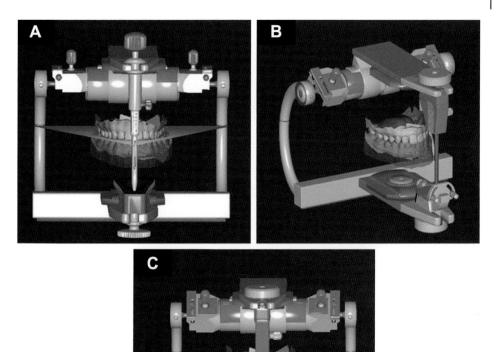

Figure 10.4 Virtual articulator mounted in the Exocad CAD software. A, Maximum intercuspal position, frontal view. B, Maximum intercuspal position, 45° view. C, Virtual incisal pin raised by 3 mm. Reproduced from Reference [7] / with permission of Taylor & Francis Group.

digital representations of the jaws and patient-specific data on jaw movement to simulate the jaw movement [11, 12]. They provide a dynamic visualization of the occlusal contacts as shown in Figure 10.4 [7]. Combined with CAD/CAM technology, this tool offers great potential in the treatment planning of prosthetic restoration since it has greater precision with a short treatment duration [11].

A facebow is an instrument used to record the spatial relationship of the maxillary arch to some anatomic reference point or points and then transfer this relationship to an articulator [5]. It orients the dental cast in the same relationship to the opening axis of the articulator. Facebow transfer is the process of transferring the facebow record of the spatial relationship of the maxillary arch and related anatomic reference points or points to an articulator (Figure 10.5).

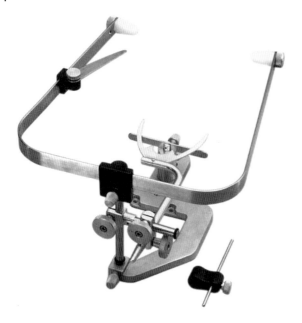

Figure 10.5 Hanau™ Spring-bow facebow.

10.3 Occlusal Concept Application Restorative Dentistry

Apart from margins and contours of a restoration, occlusal relationships play an important role in the success of dental restoration. For optimal function, the dentist must also consider two things: (i) tooth contacts and (ii) mandibular position [2].

10.3.1 Treatment Goals for Tooth Contacts

New restoration should deliver support not only to opposing teeth but also to adjacent teeth to prevent drifting or supraeruption. In addition, the new restoration must provide harmonious occlusion in posterior tooth contacts. The forces should be directed along the long axes of the teeth. Failure to attempt full reciprocation (missing an incline) may result in instability.

The anterior contacts must restore the regular form and purpose of the teeth. The anterior teeth should guide the mandible and should dislodge the posterior teeth during eccentric movements. In the closing position, the anterior teeth should contact with less force than the posterior teeth.

10.3.2 Treatment Goals for the Mandibular Position

When operative procedures are completed on a patient devoid of functional impairments, the teeth will occlude in the utmost intercuspal position (ICP). If there is any functional disorder of the masticatory system in a patient, it should be resolved before the operative procedure.

If the occlusal condition is determined to be a significant etiologic factor, selective grinding should be performed. Thus, the restorations can develop a sound occlusal relationship.

10.4 Occlusal Concept Application in Fixed Prosthodontics

Fixed prosthodontic treatments offer the advantage of adding and removing tooth surfaces till the desired restoration is precisely achieved. With the aid of articulators, restorations can be manufactured accurately, and the final adjustments can be done in the mouth. Some general guidelines for therapeutic occlusion are mentioned below [13]:

- Acceptable face height.
- Acceptable interocclusal vertical distance.
- A stable jaw relationship with bilateral contact following a relaxed closure leading to maximum intercuspation.
- Well-dispersed contacts in maximum intercuspation generating axially directed forces.
- Contact-free movements emanating from maximum intercuspation.
- No negative teeth contacts during lateral or protrusive movements.
- No soft tissue impingement with occlusal contact.

10.4.1 Treatment Goals for Tooth Contacts

The contact between the posterior teeth should deliver stability while guiding forces along the long axes of the teeth.

Appropriate axial loading can be attained by employing reciprocating incline contacts around the centric cusps (i.e. tripodization) or by establishing contact from the cusp tip to the opposing flat surface (Figures 10.6 and 10.7) [2]. Tripodization utilizes opposing tooth inclines to establish a stable intercuspal relationship. Each centric cusp is developed to have three equally distributed contacts around its tip. With some techniques, a cusp contacts an embrasure between two opposing marginal ridges, resulting in two reciprocating contacts (bipodization). A second acceptable method of developing posterior tooth

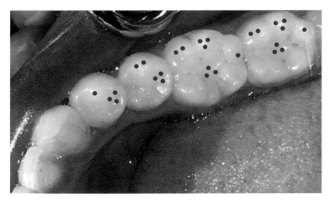

Figure 10.6 Tripodization pattern of occlusal contacts and the occlusal contacts when the areas from cusp tip to flat surface are utilized [2].

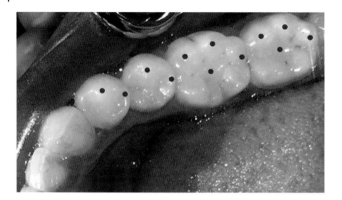

Figure 10.7 Each centric cusp contacts a fossa having three reciprocating contact areas and each centric cusp tip has a contact with a flat surface [2].

contacts is by utilizing cusp tips to flat surfaces. This allows occlusal forces to be directed through the long axes of the teeth.

The anterior teeth should make minimal contact during the closure, but substantial contact during eccentric movements. With their specific supervision pattern, fixed prosthodontic procedures permit greater regulation over the entire tooth form [2].

10.4.2 Treatment Goals for the Mandibular Position

The position of the mandible, to which fixed prosthodontic restorations are made up, is determined by two factors: (i) the existence of any functional disorder in the masticatory system, and (ii) the extent of the procedures [2].

Any functional disturbance must be treated before any fixed prosthodontic procedures. If the prevailing occlusal condition is a contributive etiologic factor, selective grinding can be performed to create a constant occlusal condition at the chosen mandibular position (CR). Once this relationship of occlusion is achieved, stable occlusal and mandibular positions are accomplished with fixed restorations.

Occlusal conditions of patients with no functional impairment are within their physiological tolerance. When a minor fixed restorative procedure (for example, a single crown) is planned, the restoration should be designed in accordance with the patient's current occlusal condition. Thus, the crown must be fabricated according to the ICP and with the existing eccentric guidance.

Nevertheless, if an extensive fixed prosthetic procedure is planned, the optimal position of the mandible (CR) must be achieved irrespective of the patient's ICP tolerance (Figure 10.8). Two factors render this suitable: The ICP is initially determined by contacts of the tooth. During the process of preparation, these contacts are removed, resulting in the loss of the original ICP. An innovative ICP is to be established with a stable position of the condyle for a stable occlusal condition. Second, this position is repeatable, which can develop a very precise occlusal condition.

Even when planning a single restoration, oral health must be considered when defining the position of the mandible for the development of the crown. The CR should be used as a reference, to achieve proper treatment goals.

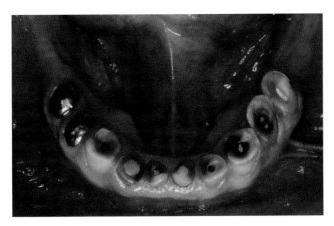

Figure 10.8 Significant wear of teeth revealing the need for significant restorative treatment. The restorative procedures must be developed in an optimal joint position.

10.5 Occlusal Concept Application in Implant Dentistry

A poor selection of occlusal schemes can result in mechanical and biological complications [14, 15]. Various complications related to dental implants are early crestal bone loss, peri-implant disease, screw loosening, implant components failure, prosthesis fracture, and porcelain fracture.

Implant-protected occlusion (IPO) addresses multiple conditions to lessen the burden on implant prostheses and bone/implant interfaces, thereby limiting implant loads within physiological limits. Proper guidelines can decrease the stresses and ensure suitable occlusal schemes to function the restoration in harmony and maximize the longevity of the implants and prostheses. The IPO allows masticatory forces within physiological limits and minimizes the occlusal overload on the prosthesis and implant/bone interface [16]. The occlusion principles for various implant prosthesis designs are shown in Table 10.1 [16].

There are various concepts regarding the functional and parafunctional demands of occlusal loading on dental implants [17]. Planning optimal occlusion schemes are an important part of implant restorations. It involves multiple interrelated factors, including satisfactory bone support, implant placement, number, length, distribution and inclination, splinting, vertical dimension, and static and dynamic occlusal schemes.

Mutual protection and anterior disclusion have acceptable therapeutic modalities in implant-supported restorations largely. Numerous variables can impact the failure of the implant and bone loss around the implant [18]. Local and general health, in addition to biomechanical factors, may be significant. The occlusion of prostheses supported by the implant can be effectively managed by employing simple procedures for the registration of the jaw and various occlusal concepts.

10.6 Occlusal Concept Application in Periodontics

Trauma from occlusion (TFO) is the injury to the periodontium resulting from occlusal forces that exceed the reparative capacity of the periodontium attachment [19, 20]. The TFO can be primary or secondary. Primary TFO is caused by the excessive occlusal force

Table 10.1 Occlusion principles for various designs of implant prosthesis. Adapted with permission from Reference [16].

Implant Prostheses	Occlusion Principles
Implant-supported fixed prosthesis	Bilateral balanced occlusion with opposing conventional complete denture.
	Group function in opposition to natural teeth.
	Infra-occlusion at the segment with a cantilevered end.
Implant-supported overdentures	Bilateral balanced occlusion with opposing conventional complete denture.
	Lingualized or one-dimensional occlusion.
Posterior implant-supported prosthesis	Anterior guidance in natural teeth.
	Group function to compromised canines.
	Cantilever reduction, occlusal table, and centralized contacts.
Single implant-supported prosthesis	Anterior guidance in natural teeth.
	Light bites concentrated contacts and strong contacts.
	Elimination of obstructions during eccentric movements.

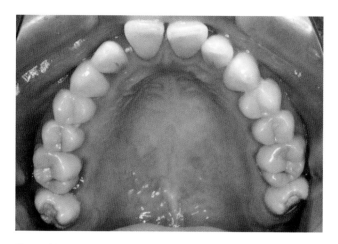

Figure 10.9 Periodontal problems in the maxillary arch (generalized bone loss, migration of anterior teeth).

exerted on a tooth or teeth with normal and healthy supporting tissues [19, 21]. Secondary TFO is the result of alterations that occur when normal or abnormal occlusal forces are delivered to a tooth or teeth with insufficient or diminished supporting tissues. Additionally, the trauma caused by occlusion can be acute or chronic [19]. Acute TFO is caused by a sudden increase in occlusal loads, such as suddenly biting on a hard object. Chronic trauma resulting from occlusion is prevalent and carries better clinical importance. Figure 10.9 shows periodontal problems in the maxillary arch (generalized bone loss, migration of anterior teeth). Mobility of the tooth is caused by several factors, which commonly include loss of attachment, loss of alveolar bone, destruction of the periodontal tissues by inflammation, heavy occlusal forces, and periodontal ligament atrophy from disuse [22].

In periodontitis, the teeth may present with various mobility buccolingually and/or vertically. The term "fremitus" refers to the mobility of the tooth during occlusal contact. It can be seen through the examiner's eyes or felt by the fingertips, or both. It may occur when the patient closes into the occlusion, or during excursions of the mandible.

For many years, TFO has been associated with periodontal disease. This does not necessarily imply that occlusal trauma is the cause of periodontitis. It implies that when occlusal loads surpass the threshold of compromised periodontal tissues, it will exacerbate pre-existing periodontal lesions. The treatment should aim to reduce occlusal forces, particularly for those with a risk of periodontitis. Tooth mobility is seen in periodontitis [22]. Clinical periodontal attachment level improved more when occlusal adjustment was incorporated into periodontal therapy. Once periodontal health has been restored, occlusal therapy can decrease mobility and restore the bone lost due to traumatic occlusal forces [23].

10.7 Occlusal Analysis and Adjustments

Occlusal adjustment is a therapy generally done by grinding teeth to produce an acceptable occlusion [24, 25]. After diagnosing the occlusal condition in the patient, the dentist needs to decide how to attain the goal of producing an acceptable occlusion without interference with harmonious function. Occlusal adjustment can be combined with other corrective measures, such as orthodontic treatment, prosthetic rehabilitation, and occlusal adjustment in clinical dentistry [24, 26].

The occlusion analysis is done by using the occlusal contact area, occlusal contact number, and occlusal force [27]. The articulating paper is a traditional, easy tool for occlusal analysis and is widely used in clinical practice. Spray powers are also available for the occlusal analysis. However, the location of occlusal contacts, size, and distribution are based on the dentist's experience and cannot be used for quantitative analysis [27, 28]. Recently, the invention of newer occlusal analysis systems, i.e. T-Scan system [29], blue silicone system [30], dental prescale system [31], and intraoral scanners (IOS) [32–34] have made quantitative analysis possible.

The developments in digital technology with dental analysis instruments have enhanced clinical success [35–39]. The IOS helps to obtain 3D digital models of the dentition [32–34], with high accuracy, patient comfort, and the possibility of a quantitative analysis [40–42]. The digital workflow and digital analysis from software allow us to measure distances, areas, and coordinates [43–45]. The digital occlusal analysis can be also done from the 3D dental model [46]. A combination of the 3D dental models obtained from IOS and quantitative data from 2D occlusal contact analysis makes it possible for quantitative analysis of occlusal contact and force simultaneously. Digital technologies use personalized jaw relation transfer and accomplish the digital duplication of the prostheses with high accuracy and less effort [42, 47].

Cao et al. [29] studied the accuracy of the 8 μm articulating paper, T-Scan system, and Cerec Omnicam system by quantitatively comparing the occlusal contacts and overlaps (Figure 10.10). The occlusal contact areas in the ICP were then quantified with Adobe Photoshop software. They found that the occlusal contacts were significantly different between the Cerec Omnicam system and the T-Scan system. The occlusal contact area

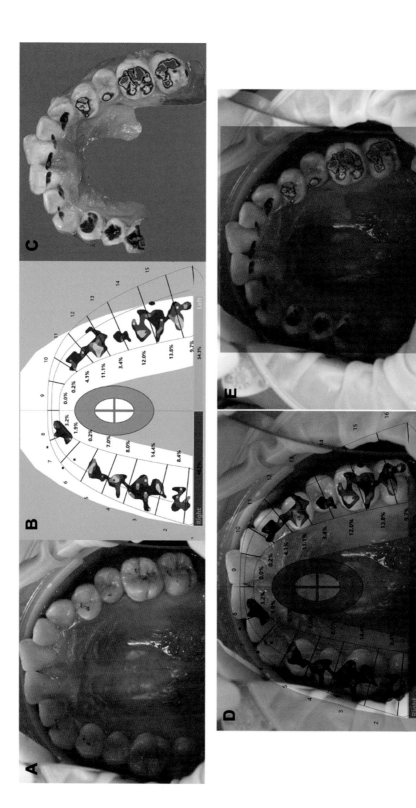

Figure 10.10 Occlusal contacts of upper left teeth measured by various tools. A, Occlusal contacts measured by T-Scan system. B, Occlusal contacts measured by Cerec Omnicam system. C, Occlusal contacts measured by articulating paper. D, Overlapping images between articulating paper and T-Scan system. E, Overlapping images between articulating paper and Cerec Omnicam system. Reproduced from Reference [29] / with permission of Elsevier.

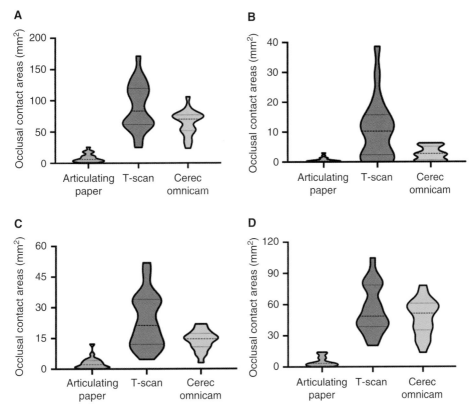

Figure 10.11 Occlusal contact area measured by articulating paper, T-Scan system, and Cerec Omnicam system. A, Anterior teeth. B, Premolars. C, Molars. D, Complete dentition. Reproduced from Reference [29] / with permission from Elsevier.

measured by the Cerec Omnicam system was smaller than that measured by the T-Scan system (Figure 10.11) [29]. The overlapping results obtained from the Cerec Omnicam system were higher than the T-Scan system. In the ICP, the accuracy of the Cerec Omnicam system for occlusal contact was higher than that of the T-Scan system, which can quantitatively analyze the occlusal relationship in terms of position, number, size, and occlusal contact points. The T-Scan system demonstrates good reproducibility in the posterior region (premolar and molar region), but poor reproducibility in the anterior teeth region.

Finally, using digital technologies such as IOS or T-Scan and 3D dental models helps with the occlusal contact analysis which makes it possible for quantitative analysis of occlusal contact and force, and visualization [29, 48].

Although digital technologies are useful diagnostic and design tools for prosthodontic and restorative care, the accuracy of these digital technologies (acquiring and analyzing) and dynamic occlusion needs further analysis [32, 49, 50]. Various factors can influence the accuracy of these digital devices. Hence, proper implementation of digital technologies into dental practice requires an understanding of the limitations and state of the current development of digital technologies and devices such as IOSs, digital jaw trackers, and computerized occlusal analysis devices.

References

1 Dawson, P.E., *Functional Occlusion: From Tmj to Smile Design*. 2006, Edinburgh: Elsevier Mosby.

2 Okeson, J.P., *Management of Temporomandibular Disorders and Occlusion*. 7th ed. 2013, St. Louis, Missouri: Mosby.

3 Mohamed, S.E., J.R. Schmidt, and J.D. Harrison, Articulators in dental education and practice. *J Prosthet Dent*, 1976. **36**(3): p. 319–325.

4 Milosevic, A., Occlusion: 3. Articulators and related instruments. *Dent Update*, 2003. **30**(9): p. 511–515.

5 Ferro K.J. The glossary of prosthodontic terms: ninth edition. *J Prosthet Dent*. 2017. **117**: p. e1–e105.

6 Rihani, A., Classification of articulators. *J Prosthet Dent*, 1980. **43**(3): p. 344–347.

7 Lin, Y.-C., R. Scialabba, J.D. Lee, J. Sun, and S.J. Lee, Assessment of occlusal vertical dimension change in mechanical and virtual articulation: a pilot study. *Dent J*, 2022. **10**(11): p. 212.

8 Koralakunte, P.R. and M. Aljanakh, The role of virtual articulator in prosthetic and restorative dentistry. *J Clin Diagn Res*, 2014. **8**(7): p. Ze25–Ze28.

9 Kordass, B., C. Gärtner, A. Söhnel, A. Bisler, G. Voss, U. Bockholt, and S. Seipel, The virtual articulator in dentistry: concept and development. *Dent Clin N Am*, 2002. **46**(3): p. 493–506, vi.

10 Maestre-Ferrín, L., J. Romero-Millán, D. Peñarrocha-Oltra, and M. Peñarrocha-Diago, Virtual articulator for the analysis of dental occlusion: an update. *Med Oral Patol Oral Cir Bucal*, 2012. **17**(1): p. e160–e163.

11 Bisler, A., U. Bockholt, B. Kordass, M. Suchan, and G. Voss, The virtual articulator. *Int J Comput Dent*, 2002. **5**(2–3): p. 101–106.

12 Lepidi, L., M. Galli, F. Mastrangelo, P. Venezia, T. Joda, H.L. Wang, and J. Li, Virtual articulators and virtual mounting procedures: where do we stand? *J Prosthodont*, 2021. **30**(1): p. 24–35.

13 Tangerud, T. and G.E. Carlsson, Jaw registration and occlusal morphology, in *A Textbook of Fixed Prosthodontics. The Scandinavian Approach*, S. Karlsson, K. Nilner, and B.L. Dahl, Editors. 2000, Gothia: Stockholm. p. 209–230.

14 Verma, M., A. Nanda, and A. Sood, Principles of occlusion in implant dentistry. *J Int Clin Dent Res Organ*, 2015. **7**(3): p. 27–33.

15 Chen, Y.Y., C.L. Kuan, and Y.B. Wang, Implant occlusion: biomechanical considerations for implant supported prostheses. *J Dent Sci*, 2008. **3**: p. 65–74.

16 Oliveira, A., A. Bessa, and F. Dias, Clinical applications of occlusion principles in implantology - narrative review. *JSPIR*, 2019. **1**: p. 40–45.

17 Gross, M.D., Occlusion in implant dentistry. A review of the literature of prosthetic determinants and current concepts. *Aust Dent J*, 2008. **53** Suppl 1: p. S60–S68.

18 Carlsson, G.E., Dental occlusion: modern concepts and their application in implant prosthodontics. *Odontology*, 2009. **97**(1): p. 8–17.

19 Davies, S.J., R.J. Gray, G.J. Linden, and J.A. James, Occlusal considerations in periodontics. *Br Dent J*, 2001. **191**(11): p. 597–604.

20 Wank, G.S. and Y.J. Kroll, Occlusal trauma. An evaluation of its relationship to periodontal prostheses. *Dent Clin N Am*, 1981. **25**(3): p. 511–532.

21 Sanz, M., Occlusion in a periodontal context. *Int J Prosthodont*, 2005. **18**(4): p. 309–310.

22 Gher, M.E., Changing concepts. The effects of occlusion on periodontitis. *Dent Clin N Am*, 1998. **42**(2): p. 285–299.

23 Serio, F.G. and C.E. Hawley, Periodontal trauma and mobility. Diagnosis and treatment planning. *Dent Clin N Am*, 1999. **43**(1): p. 37–44.

24 Carlsson, G.E., Occlusal adjustment by grinding of teeth; indications and techniques. *Rev Belge Med Dent*, 1976. **31**(2): p. 143–151.

25 Oles, R.D., Occlusal adjustment. *J Can Dent Assoc*, 1990. **56**(6): p. 527–531.

26 Gray, H.S., Occlusal adjustment: principles and practice. *N Z Dent J*, 1994. **90**(399): p. 13–19.

27 Zhao, Z., Q. Wang, J. Li, M. Zhou, K. Tang, J. Chen, and F. Wang, Construction of a novel digital method for quantitative analysis of occlusal contact and force. *BMC Oral Health*, 2023. **23**(1): p. 190.

28 Majithia, I.P., V. Arora, S. Anil Kumar, V. Saxena, and M. Mittal, Comparison of articulating paper markings and T Scan III recordings to evaluate occlusal force in normal and rehabilitated maxillofacial trauma patients. *Med J Armed Forces India*, 2015. **71**(Suppl 2): p. S382–S388.

29 Cao, R., H. Xu, J. Lin, and W. Liu, Evaluation of the accuracy of T-scan system and Cerec Omnicam system used in occlusal contact assessment. *Heliyon*, 2023. **9**(2): p. e13476.

30 Okada, Y., Y. Sato, N. Kitagawa, K. Uchida, T. Osawa, Y. Imamura, and M. Terazawa, Occlusal status of implant superstructures at mandibular first molar immediately after setting. *Int J Implant Dent*, 2015. **1**(1): p. 16.

31 Shiga, H., M. Komino, H. Uesugi, M. Sano, M. Yokoyama, K. Nakajima, and A. Ishikawa, Comparison of two dental prescale systems used for the measurement of occlusal force. *Odontology*, 2020. **108**(4): p. 676–680.

32 Revilla-León, M., D.E. Kois, J.M. Zeitler, W. Att, and J.C. Kois, An overview of the digital occlusion technologies: intraoral scanners, jaw tracking systems, and computerized occlusal analysis devices. *J Esthet Restor Dent*, 2023. **35**(5): p. 735–744.

33 Hou, C., H.Z. Zhu, B. Xue, H.J. Song, Y.B. Yang, X.X. Wang, and H.Q. Sun, New clinical application of digital intraoral scanning technology in occlusal reconstruction: a case report. *World J Clin Cases*, 2023. **11**(15): p. 3522–3532.

34 Michou, S., C. Vannahme, A. Bakhshandeh, K.R. Ekstrand, and A.R. Benetti, Intraoral scanner featuring transillumination for proximal caries detection. An in vitro validation study on permanent posterior teeth. *J Dent*, 2022. **116**: p. 103841.

35 Humagain, M. and D. Rokaya, Integrating digital technologies in dentistry to enhance the clinical success. *Kathmandu Univ Med J (KUMJ)*, 2019. **17**(68): p. 256–257.

36 McBeath, K.C.C., C.E. Angermann, and M.R. Cowie, Digital technologies to support better outcome and experience of care in patients with heart failure. *Curr Heart Fail Rep*, 2022. **19**(3): p. 75–108.

37 Giese-Kraft, K., K. Jung, N. Schlueter, K. Vach, and C. Ganss, Detecting and monitoring dental plaque levels with digital 2D and 3D imaging techniques. *PLoS One*, 2022. **17**(2): p. e0263722.

38 Woodsend, B., E. Koufoudaki, P. Lin, G. McIntyre, A. El-Angbawi, A. Aziz, W. Shaw, G. Semb, G.V. Reesu, and P.A. Mossey, Development of intra-oral automated landmark recognition (ALR) for dental and occlusal outcome measurements. *Eur J Orthod*, 2022. **44**(1): p. 43–50.

39 Lahoud, P., R. Jacobs, P. Boisse, M. EzEldeen, M. Ducret, and R. Richert, Precision medicine using patient-specific modelling: state of the art and perspectives in dental practice. *Clin Oral Investig*, 2022. **26**(8): p. 5117–5128.

40 Michelinakis, G., D. Apostolakis, A. Tsagarakis, G. Kourakis, and E. Pavlakis, A comparison of accuracy of 3 intraoral scanners: a single-blinded in vitro study. *J Prosthet Dent*, 2020. **124**(5): p. 581–588.

41 Rajshekar, M., R. Julian, A.M. Williams, M. Tennant, A. Forrest, L.J. Walsh, G. Wilson, and L. Blizzard, The reliability and validity of measurements of human dental casts made by an intra-oral 3D scanner, with conventional hand-held digital callipers as the comparison measure. *Forensic Sci Int*, 2017. **278**: p. 198–204.

42 Kim, J.E., J.H. Park, H.S. Moon, and J.S. Shim, Complete assessment of occlusal dynamics and establishment of a digital workflow by using target tracking with a three-dimensional facial scanner. *J Prosthodont Res*, 2019. **63**(1): p. 120–124.

43 Marques, S., P. Ribeiro, C. Gama, and M. Herrero-Climent, Digital guided veneer preparation: a dental technique. *J Prosthet Dent*, 2022. https://doi.org/10.1016/j.prosdent.2022.04.035 (In Press).

44 Conejo, J., S. Han, P.J. Atria, L. Stone-Hirsh, J. Dubin, and M.B. Blatz, Full digital workflow to resolve angled adjacent dental implants: a dental technique. *J Prosthet Dent*, 2022. https://doi.org/10.1016/j.prosdent.2022.07.012 (Online ahead of print).

45 Kongkiatkamon, S. and D. Rokaya, Full digital workflow in the esthetic dental restoration. *Case Rep Dent*, 2022. **2022**: p. 8836068.

46 Ayuso-Montero, R., Y. Mariano-Hernandez, L. Khoury-Ribas, B. Rovira-Lastra, E. Willaert, and J. Martinez-Gomis, Reliability and validity of T-scan and 3D intraoral scanning for measuring the occlusal contact area. *J Prosthodont*, 2020. **29**(1): p. 19–25.

47 Wang, J., C. Jin, B. Dong, L. Yue, and S. Gao, Fully digital workflow for replicating treatment dentures: a technique for jaw relation transfer and dynamic occlusal adjustment. *J Prosthet Dent*, 2023. **130**(3): p. 288–294.

48 Solaberrieta, E., J.R. Otegi, N. Goicoechea, A. Brizuela, and G. Pradies, Comparison of a conventional and virtual occlusal record. *J Prosthet Dent*, 2015. **114**(1): p. 92–97.

49 Revilla-León, M., L. Fernández-Estevan, A.B. Barmak, J.C. Kois, and J.A. Pérez-Barquero, Accuracy of the maxillomandibular relationship at centric relation position recorded by using 3 different intraoral scanners with or without an optical jaw tracking system: an in vivo pilot study. *J Dent*, 2023. **132**: p. 104478.

50 Revilla-León, M., R. Agustín-Panadero, J.M. Zeitler, A.B. Barmak, B. Yilmaz, J.C. Kois, and J.A. Pérez-Barquero, Differences in maxillomandibular relationship recorded at centric relation when using a conventional method, four intraoral scanners, and a jaw tracking system: a clinical study. *J Prosthet Dent*, 2023. https://doi.org/10.1016/j.prosdent.2022.12.007 (Online ahead of print).

11

Problems in Occlusion

11.1 Introduction

The problems of occlusion can be tooth surface loss, limited interocclusal space crack/ fracturing of teeth, and occlusal trauma. [1]. According to Lytle, occlusal disease is the process leading to the destruction of the occlusal surfaces of the teeth [2]. The occlusal disease may cause occlusal problems. The destruction of the occlusal surface of teeth results from the following three mechanisms [3].

1) Occlusal stress resulting in tension, compression, and flexure can result in microfracture and abfraction of teeth.
2) Abrasion from exogenous material and attrition from endogenous causes (bruxing and parafunction habits). Both result in teeth wear.
3) Corrosion from chemical or electrochemical degradation.

Attrition is caused by tooth-to-tooth contact and results in wear facets on the occluding posterior teeth [1]. Physiological tooth wear occurs to a certain level according to the age of the patient. Further, wear results in pathological tooth wear because of parafunctional activity, compromises the pulp health, and often results in the loss of interocclusal space causing difficulty in the correction and restoration of interocclusal relationships [4].

Temporomandibular joint disorder (TMD) is a multifactorial disease, and occlusal disharmony is a major predisposing factor [1, 5, 6]. The dental-related risk factors of TMD are >5 mm overjet, intercuspal position slides of >1.75 mm, posterior crossbite, and retruded contact position [5].

11.2 Complete Dentistry

A complete dental examination identifies all factors contributing to the deterioration of oral health or function. It is the responsibility of the examiner to examine signs of deterioration before they cause symptoms. The seven goals for patient care are as follows, and they result in the foundation for complete dentistry [7]:

1) Free from masticatory apparatus diseases.
2) Healthy teeth.

Introduction to the Masticatory System and Dental Occlusion, First Edition. Dinesh Rokaya.
© 2025 John Wiley & Sons Ltd. Published 2025 by John Wiley & Sons Ltd.

3) Healthy periodontium.
4) Stable occlusion.
5) Stable TMJs.
6) Comfortable function.
7) Optimum esthetics.

11.3 Treatment of Occlusal Problems

It is important to identify the parafunctional activity before treatment at the planning stages to protect the tooth structure and restoration. The treatment strategies for the occlusal problems are shown below [1].

- Tooth surface loss: They present wear facets, short teeth, or dentine sensitivity. They can be treated by preventive and splint therapy or restorations with increased vertical dimensions.
- Tooth surface loss with less interocclusal space: They present limited space for restorations. They can be treated by the Dahl technique, crown lengthening, or intrusion orthodontically.
- Crack/fracture of teeth: They generally have large restorations with less tooth structure support. They can be treated with cuspal coverage restorations (onlay or crown).
- Occlusal trauma: Occlusal trauma exacerbates periodontal disease. Management of periodontal disease should be done with occlusal adjustment.
- TMD from occlusion: They present with pain of masticatory muscles and TMJ, wear or facet, and TMJ clicking. They can be treated with occlusal adjustment, stress reduction, TMJ exercises, and patient education.

11.3.1 Accomplishing Treatment Goals in Operative Dentistry

Examination of the occlusion to the operative procedure helps to accomplish the treatment goals. This can be done by examination of the diagnostic casts or in patients by using articulating paper or digital methods. Locating the existing contacts can help in restoring these contacts on the restored teeth.

11.3.1.1 Contacts in Anterior Teeth

In anterior restorations, tooth morphology is an important aspect. When the composite is completed, the occlusion must be evaluated. Heavy contact tends to cause vibration (i.e. fremitus) or may displace the teeth labially and they should be reduced [1]. After adjusting the contacts during the closure of the mandible, the eccentric movements are evaluated. If the eccentric pathway is noted, it should be adjusted to provide smooth movement.

11.3.1.2 Contacts in Posterior Teeth

It can be a difficult task to restore the stable posterior tooth contacts on new restorations. A new amalgam restoration with increased or excessive height can lead to a fracture of the restoration, whereas, a new composite restoration with excessive height can lead to discomfort or pain in teeth while biting. Sometimes, the patients cannot detect some alteration in the occlusion following restorations and can develop unstable occlusion from drifting of the teeth to establish a new occlusal contact. This can result in undesirable occlusal relationships or eccentric contacts (Figure 11.1).

The amalgam or composite restoration should be carved into using articulating paper and should be out of occlusion. By checking occlusion prior to operative procedure and restoration, one can gain an idea of the extent of carving needed. After proper ICP is established, the eccentric contacts are evaluated – straight protrusive, laterotrusive movements, and various lateroprotrusive excursions. As in selective grinding, the colored markings can be helpful in locating the eccentric contacts during closure. Generally, amalgam or

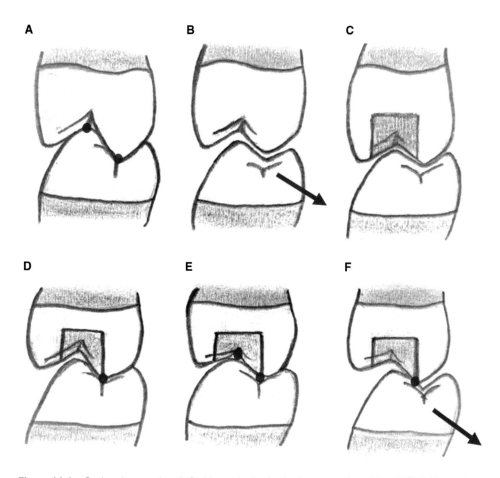

Figure 11.1 Occlusal correction. A, Stable occlusion in the intercuspal position (ICP). B, No teeth contact during a mediotrusive movement. C, Tooth preparation on the maxillary molar. D, An over-contoured amalgam restoration resulting in no contact of buccal cusps. E, The mandibular tooth re-establishes contact between the cusp (buccal) and the restoration to create a stable occlusion after some time. F, A mediotrusive contact has resulted although with stable ICP. Adapted from Reference [7]; chapter published in Management of Temporomandibular Disorders and Occlusion, 7th edition, Okeson J.P., Restorative Considerations in Occlusal Therapy, page 457, Copyright Elsevier (2013).

composite restorations should not be used as guidance for the movement of the mandible, hence, eccentric contact should be eliminated on the restorations.

11.3.2 Accomplishing Treatment Goals in Fixed Prosthodontics

In fixed prosthetic treatments, it is important to develop the anterior tooth contacts for acceptable guidance during eccentric mandibular movements.

11.3.2.1 Contacts in Anterior Teeth

Examination of the occlusal relationships of the anterior teeth should be done before starting any prosthodontic treatments. The adequate anterior guidance should be determined with the extent of disocclusion of the posterior teeth. The morphology of the anterior teeth provides anterior guidance. During the teeth preparation, the existing guidance is obliterated. Once the new restorations are fabricated arbitrarily, the guidance of such produce is less tolerated by the patient. New less steep anterior guidance may not disocclude the posterior teeth during the eccentric movement. Similarly, new too steep anterior guidance may restrict mandibular pattern which can compromise muscle function. Hence, precise anterior guidance should be maintained and preserved. The anterior guidance characteristics can be recorded and preserved on a semiadjustable articulator by the custom anterior guidance table. The provisional restorations with new anterior guidance can be given for several weeks to a few months to determine comfort and acceptance. The provisional is altered accordingly until acceptable guidance is attained. When suitable guidance is achieved, diagnostic casts of the teeth can be made and mounted on the articulator. Then, the final restoration can be proceeded with a custom anterior guidance table.

11.3.2.2 Contacts in Posterior Teeth

After achieving adequate anterior guidance, the posterior teeth can be restored to provide stable occlusion in the CR position. The posterior contacts should contact occlusion and direct occlusal forces through the long axes of the teeth. This can be obtained from a tripodization contact pattern for the centric cusps, or by contact from the centric cusp tip to a flat surface (as described in Chapter 10). Each technique has advantages and disadvantages. Tripodization is useful in full reconstruction although it is difficult to achieve. Stable occlusion is also achieved with a technique of cusp tip to the flat surface. Furthermore, the cusp-fossa relationship lends to these techniques.

11.3.3 Selective Grinding

Selective grinding is a technique to accurately alter the occlusal surfaces of the teeth to improve contact. In this procedure, tooth structure from the occlusal surface is selectively removed to contact the teeth to fulfill the treatment goals. This procedure can be used to manage certain occlusal problems as in TMD and help the treatment associated with major occlusal changes. For TMD patients, apart from occlusal adjustment and splint therapy, patient education with jaw exercises provides significant improvements [8].

Another way is the elimination of the CR slide. A mandible slide results from unstable contacts on tooth inclines in opposing teeth. Thus, the treatment goal is to achieve acceptable contacts in ICP by altering or reshaping the cuspal inclines. A cusp tip to flat surface relationship is desirable as no shift occurs in this relation.

Figures 11.2–11.4 show the selective grinding sequence in CR. When a contact is found on an incline close to a centric cusp tip (Figure 11.2A), it is eliminated to create posterior teeth that come together [7]. The contact area will be shifted up closer to the cusp tip (Figures 11.2B, D, 11.3B, D, 11.4A, B). When a contact area is located on the incline near the central fossa, the incline should be reshaped into a flat surface. This technique is often called hollow grinding (Figures 11.2D, 11.3D, 11.4C, and 11.4D) [7]. These alterations will result in proper tooth contact (Figures 11.2C, 11.3E, and 11.4D).

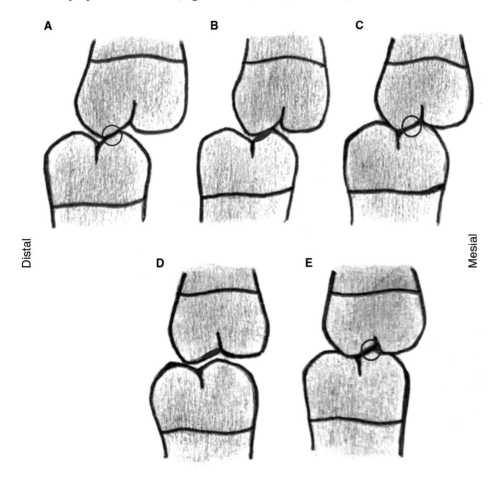

Figure 11.2 Selective grinding in centric relation (buccal view) to achieve proper contacts between maxillary and mandibular teeth during closure. A, The mesial incline of the maxillary tooth contacts the distal incline of the mandibular tooth in centric relation. B, Elimination of the incline in the mandibular tooth to allow the cusp tip to contact. C, After the correction, the mandibular cusp tip contacts the mesial incline of a maxillary cusp during closure. D, This incline is reshaped into a flat surface (hollow grinding) in the maxillary tooth. E, After the correction, the mandibular cusp tip contacts the maxillary flat surface of the maxillary tooth. Adapted from Reference [7]; chapter published in Management of Temporomandibular Disorders and Occlusion, 7th edition, Okeson J.P., Selective Grinding, page 447, Copyright Elsevier (2013).

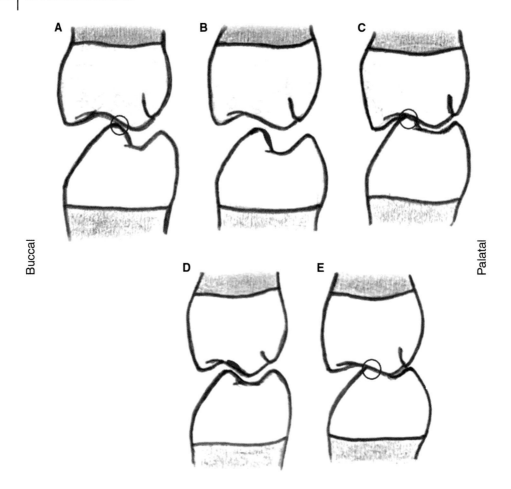

Buccal

Palatal

Figure 11.3 Selective grinding in centric relation (mesial view) to achieve proper contacts between maxillary and mandibular teeth during closure. A, The inner incline of the maxillary tooth contacts the inner incline of the mandibular tooth in centric relation. B, Elimination of the incline in the mandibular tooth to allow the cusp tip to contact. C, After the correction, the mandibular cusp tip contacts the inner incline of the maxillary centric cusp during closure. D, This incline is reshaped into a flat surface (hollow grinding) in the maxillary tooth. E, After the correction, the mandibular cusp tip contacts the flat surface of the maxillary tooth. Adapted from Reference [7]; chapter published in Management of Temporomandibular Disorders and Occlusion, 7th edition, Okeson J.P., Selective Grinding, page 447, Copyright Elsevier (2013).

Once the desirable guidance contacts have been defined, the eccentric contacts are eliminated. For this, two different marking papers (red and blue) are used [7]. All eccentric contacts consisting of protrusive, laterotrusive, and mediotrusive are marked blue and the CR contacts are marked red. Then, the eccentric contacts can be adjusted without altering red CR contacts. A red dot with a blue streak extending from it is generally seen (Figure 11.5) [7]. It shows that the centric cusp tip contacts the tooth incline in opposing teeth during an eccentric movement.

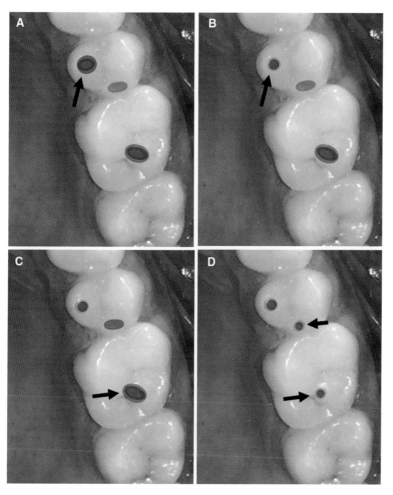

Figure 11.4 Selective grinding. A, In centric relation, tooth contact occurs on the inner incline and cusp tip of the maxillary second premolar. B, The contact area is altered to contact only the cusp tip contacts. C, In centric relation, a contact occurs on the incline near the central fossa of this maxillary first molar. D, The contact area is altered into a flat surface (hollow grinding) to make contact on the marginal ridge of the second premolar.

After completing the selective grinding procedure, the cusp tips and flat surfaces show centric relation (CR) contacts. Canines and premolars show only laterotrusive contacts with no mediotrusive contacts [7]. The incisors also present blue protrusive contacts (Figure 11.6). Following selective grinding, group function guidance can be developed.

Correct diagnosis is important in the management of occlusal problems. Occlusal splints are used to treat occlusal problems. Figure 11.7 shows the patient with abraded teeth surfaces from bruxism [9]. At present, various digital technologies are used in clinical dentistry for oral rehabilitation and occlusal adjustments [10–12]. Figure 11.8 shows the use of digital technologies (intraoral scan and software) to fabricate a splint and 3D with clear resin. A 2.7 mm thick occlusal splint was fabricated, and the T-Scan Novus system was used

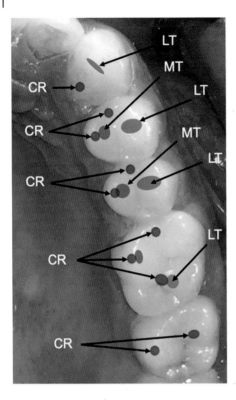

Figure 11.5 Red markings are used for the centric relation (CR) contacts and blue markings are used for the eccentric contacts; laterotrusive (LT) and mediotrusive (MT). Reproduced from Reference [7] / Okeson et.al., / Elsevier; chapter published in Management of Temporomandibular Disorders and Occlusion, 7th edition, Okeson J.P., Selective Grinding, page 452, Copyright Elsevier (2013).

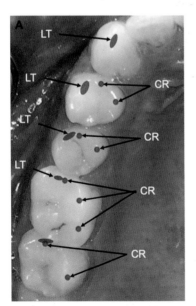

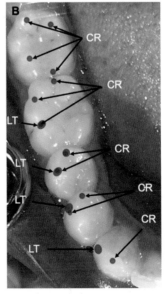

Figure 11.6 Selective grinding completed in the maxillary and mandibular arch (right side). A, Maxillary teeth. B, Mandibular teeth.

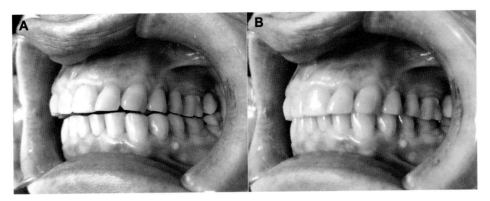

Figure 11.7 Patient showing an occlusal problem. A, Disocclusion of the maxillary arch and mandibular arch showing abraded teeth. B, Centric occlusion. Reproduced from Reference [9] / with permission of Journal of Orthopaedic & Sports Physical Therapy (JOSPT).

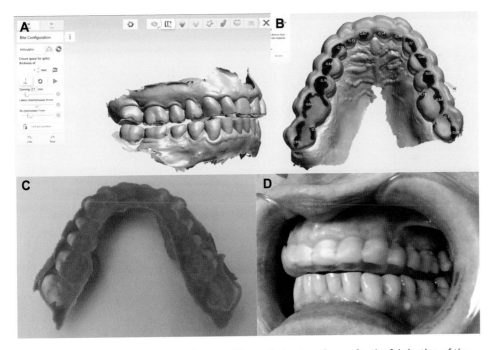

Figure 11.8 Fabrication of splint. A, Intermaxillary relation in software for the fabrication of the splint. B, Balanced occlusion from software. C, Silicone bite. D, Fabricated splint in the patient's mouth. Reproduced from Reference [9] / with permission of Journal of Orthopaedic & Sports Physical Therapy (JOSPT).

for the digital examination of the occlusion Figure 11.9. The position of the TMJ components was proven radiologically. It showed that using digital technology allows for more accurate constructions and precise balancing of occlusal relationships.

Finally, it has been shown that the use of digital technologies allows more precise examination, visualization, and fabrication of the occlusal splints and dental adaptation of the

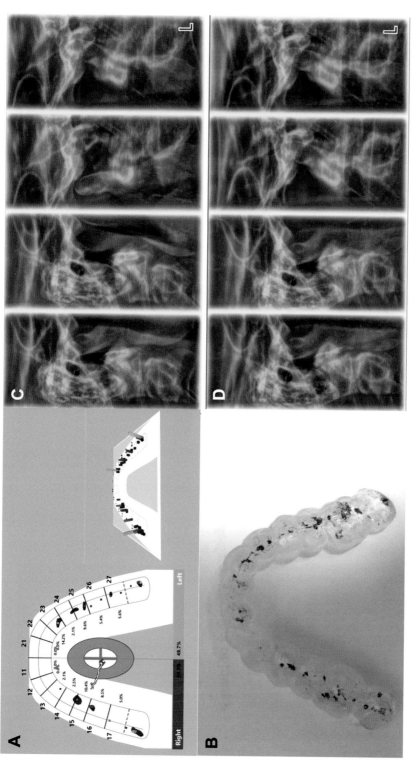

Figure 11.9 Occlusal correction and adjustment. A, Final occlusal registration in the T-scan software. B, Final occlusal registration in the splint. C, Condyles position (open and closed) before splint fabrication. D, Condyles position (open and closed) after the splint in the patient's mouth. Reproduced from Reference [9] / with permission of Journal of Orthopaedic & Sports Physical Therapy (JOSPT).

splint, occlusal relief, and occlusal relationships [13–15]. Digital workflow techniques have advantages compared with traditional methods, including a jaw motion analyzer and virtual articulator to transfer jaw relations, which ensures accurate maxillomandibular relationships and a balanced occlusion [13, 16–18]. In addition, the digital workflow simplifies the manufacturing process and requires less human input reducing the risk of infection, and the technique avoids errors, including cast deformation, errors in articulator settings, and acrylic resin deformation.

Although digital technologies are useful diagnostic and design tools for prosthodontic and restorative care, the accuracy of these digital technologies (acquiring and analyzing) and dynamic occlusion needs further analysis [19–21]. Various factors can influence the accuracy of these digital devices. Hence, proper implementation of digital technologies into dental practice requires an understanding of the limitations and state of the current development of digital technologies and devices such as IOSs, digital jaw trackers, and computerized occlusal analysis devices.

References

1 Alani, A. and M. Patel, Clinical issues in occlusion – part I. *Singap Dent J*, 2014. **35**: p. 31–38.

2 Lytle, J.D., Clinician's index of occlusal disease: definition, recognition, and management. *Int J Periodontics Restorative Dent*, 1990. **10**(2): p. 102–123.

3 Grippo, J.O., M. Simring, and S. Schreiner, Attrition, abrasion, corrosion and abfraction revisited: a new perspective on tooth surface lesions. *J Am Dent Assoc*, 2004. **135**(8): p. 1109–1118.

4 Dawson, P.E., *Functional Occlusion: From Tmj to Smile Design*. 2006, Edinburgh: Elsevier Mosby.

5 Dzingutė, A., G. Pileičikienė, A. Baltrušaitytė, and G. Skirbutis, Evaluation of the relationship between the occlusion parameters and symptoms of the temporomandibular joint disorder. *Acta Medica Lituanica*, 2017. **24**(3): p. 167–175.

6 Pullinger, A.G. and D.A. Seligman, Quantification and validation of predictive values of occlusal variables in temporomandibular disorders using a multifactorial analysis. *J Prosthet Dent*, 2000. **83**(1): p. 66–75.

7 Okeson, J.P., *Management of Temporomandibular Disorders and Occlusion*. 7th ed. 2013, St. Louis, Missouri: Mosby.

8 McNeill, C., Management of temporomandibular disorders: concepts and controversies. *J Prosthet Dent*, 1997. **77**(5): p. 510–522.

9 Shopova, D., T. Bozhkova, S. Yordanova, and M. Yordanova, Case report: digital analysis of occlusion with T-Scan Novus in occlusal splint treatment for a patient with bruxism. *F1000Res*, 2021. **10**: 915.

10 Peng, T., Z. Yang, T. Ma, M. Zhang, and G. Ren, Comparative evaluation of the volume of occlusal adjustment of repositioning occlusal devices designed by using an average value digital articulator and the jaw movement analyzer. *J Prosthet Dent*, 2023. https://doi.org/10.1016/j.prosdent.2023.06.018 (Online ahead of print).

11 McBeath, K.C.C., C.E. Angermann, and M.R. Cowie, Digital technologies to support better outcome and experience of care in patients with heart failure. *Curr Heart Fail Rep*, 2022. **19**(3): p. 75–108.

12 Humagain, M. and D. Rokaya, Integrating digital technologies in dentistry to enhance the clinical success. *Kathmandu Univ Med J (KUMJ)*, 2019. **17**(68): p. 256–257.

13 Solaberrieta, E., J.R. Otegi, N. Goicoechea, A. Brizuela, and G. Pradies, Comparison of a conventional and virtual occlusal record. *J Prosthet Dent*, 2015. **114**(1): p. 92–97.

14 Stavness, I.K., A.G. Hannam, D.L. Tobias, and X. Zhang, Simulation of dental collisions and occlusal dynamics in the virtual environment. *J Oral Rehabil*, 2016. **43**(4): p. 269–278.

15 Krahenbuhl, J.T., S.H. Cho, J. Irelan, and N.K. Bansal, Accuracy and precision of occlusal contacts of stereolithographic casts mounted by digital interocclusal registrations. *J Prosthet Dent*, 2016. **116**(2): p. 231–236.

16 Wang, J., C. Jin, B. Dong, L. Yue, and S. Gao, Fully digital workflow for replicating treatment dentures: a technique for jaw relation transfer and dynamic occlusal adjustment. *J Prosthet Dent*, 2023. **130**(3): p. 288–294.

17 Kim, J.E., J.H. Park, H.S. Moon, and J.S. Shim, Complete assessment of occlusal dynamics and establishment of a digital workflow by using target tracking with a three-dimensional facial scanner. *J Prosthodont Res*, 2019. **63**(1): p. 120–124.

18 Kongkiatkamon, S. and D. Rokaya, Full digital workflow in the esthetic dental restoration. *Case Rep Dent*, 2022. **2022**: p. 8836068.

19 Revilla-León, M., D.E. Kois, J.M. Zeitler, W. Att, and J.C. Kois, An overview of the digital occlusion technologies: intraoral scanners, jaw tracking systems, and computerized occlusal analysis devices. *J Esthet Restor Dent*, 2023. **35**(5): p. 735–744.

20 Revilla-León, M., L. Fernández-Estevan, A.B. Barmak, J.C. Kois, and J.A. Pérez-Barquero, Accuracy of the maxillomandibular relationship at centric relation position recorded by using 3 different intraoral scanners with or without an optical jaw tracking system: an in vivo pilot study. *J Dent*, 2023. **132**: p. 104478.

21 Revilla-León, M., R. Agustín-Panadero, J.M. Zeitler, A.B. Barmak, B. Yilmaz, J.C. Kois, and J.A. Pérez-Barquero, Differences in maxillomandibular relationship recorded at centric relation when using a conventional method, four intraoral scanners, and a jaw tracking system: A clinical study. *J Prosthet Dent*, 2023. https://doi.org/10.1016/j.prosdent.2022.12.007 (Online ahead of print).

Index

a

abrasion   50, 159
adaptive changes   135
aging   43, 116–118, 133–139
anterior guidance   42, 47–49, 55–58, 66, 129, 152, 162
arch circumference   25
arch form   22–23, 27
arch length   24–25, 32
arch width   17, 23–25
attrition   124, 159
awake bruxism   121, 122, 125

b

Bennet's angle   60
Bennett's movement   60
bipodization   149
body planes   68, 69, 146
border movements   44, 55, 73–83, 129
brain   103, 109, 110, 115
brainstem   90, 109
bruxism   15, 82, 121–130, 165
buccal embrasure   28, 29
bucco-occlusal line   27–28

c

canine guidance   42, 46, 49–50, 91
canine relationship   42
capsular ligament   3, 74
central fossa   36, 39, 42, 163, 165
central fossa line   27–28
central pattern generator   87
centric bruxism   129

centric cusp   27–29, 65, 149–150, 162–164
centric occlusion   30, 36, 44–47, 76, 80, 82, 91, 149, 167
centric stop   36, 51
cervical muscles   14, 110
chewing stroke   17, 29, 76, 88–89, 91–93, 101
clenching   14, 15, 121–130
collateral ligaments   2–3
complete dentistry   159–160
condylar guidance   54–56, 66, 69, 73
contact areas   28–30, 41, 50, 150, 153–155, 163, 165
corrosion   159
cortex   108–110
crushing   17, 88, 91–92
curve of Spee   25–26, 57–60
curve of Wilson   25–26
cusp height   56–63

d

deglutition   83, 94, 138
dental occlusion   36–37, 68
dentation   135–136
digastric   14, 15, 89

e

electromyography   129, 135
emotional stress   129
envelope of motion   68, 80–82

f

fixed prosthodontics   144, 149–151, 162
flexor reflex   114–115

Introduction to the Masticatory System and Dental Occlusion, First Edition. Dinesh Rokaya.
© 2025 John Wiley & Sons Ltd. Published 2025 by John Wiley & Sons Ltd.